Exercise for Better Bones

The Complete Guide to Safe and Effective Exercises for Osteoporosis

Margaret Martin, PT, CSCS

Exercise for Better Bones

The Complete Guide to Safe and Effective Exercises for Osteoporosis.

Copyright © 2016 by Margaret Martin.

Photography: Richard Martin

Interior Design: Richard Martin

Video Production: Richard Martin

Published in Canada by Kamajojo Press.

ISBN-13: 978-0991912544

ISBN-10: 0991912543

Version 4.1

Find us on the Web at www.melioguide.com

To report errors, please send a note to info@melioguide.com

Exercise for Better Bones
Table of Contents

Acknowledgements

The development of my website, the professional workshops, the online professional training courses, and this guide were made possible by the tireless support from, encouragement of, and thousands of hours of skilled labor by my husband, Richard.

This guide is dedicated to my many clients who were initially fearful of moving and breaking a bone when they were first told that they had osteoporosis. Helping them build their confidence and strength motivated me to reach out to others with similar challenges. Their questions helped me become a better Therapist.

I would especially like to acknowledge my clients who posed for earlier versions of the manual and website, especially Aline Young and Pat Heydon for their willingness to sit through the revised version of the site and guide. I thank them for their time, their patience, and their unending smiles.

I need to acknowledge the contributions of all the Physical Therapists, Physiotherapists, Occupational Therapists, Kinesiologists, and other health care professionals that I have had the privilege of training around the world – both online and live workshops. Your feedback and recommendations have improved the site, this manual, and my books. I would especially like to thank Holly Bonasera and Betsey Newcomb for reviewing early drafts of this guide and Marian Weldon and Karen Kemmis for their support and encouragement during the early stages of this project. A "thank you" to Sara Meeks for teaching me the importance of posture and alignment in the treatment of osteoporosis.

Hundreds of researchers have studied the effects of exercise on bone. Without their dedication and perseverance, we would not understand the benefits and risks of exercise. To the Doctors of Physical Therapy, Kathy Shipp at Duke University, Meena Sran at University of British Columbia, and Wendy Katzman at University of California in San Franscisco, thank you for your support and feedback during the development of MelioGuide.

Lastly, to our children, John and Katherine, who claim to be the only Millenials who know everything there is to know about building stronger bones. Thank you for letting us spill out our ideas and excitement around the house and cottage.

Margaret Martin

Physical Therapist, Certified Strength and Conditioning Specialist

July, 2015

Ottawa, Canada

1. Welcome

Congratulations! You have made a significant step towards building healthier, stronger bones and reducing your risk of a fracture. I am looking forward to working with you as you build both your bones and your confidence!

Medical research has shown over and over again that exercise is a critical component in building and maintaining strong bones and reducing the risk of a fracture[1,2]. The research and scientific data supporting the benefits of exercise on bones is quite convincing.

I find the positive results of a well-designed bone building exercise program on clients at my Physiotherapy clinic to be very motivating. I hope that you experience the same level of excitement, achievement, and confidence as you follow the Exercise for Better Bones program in this guide.

I am fortunate to work with all kinds of people and watch them build their confidence as they develop their strength, balance, flexibility, and cardiovascular endurance, and improve their posture. In addition to developing exercise programs appropriate to their fracture risk and activity level, I also teach them that everyday activities and positions can lead to a fracture and, as a result, would best be modified. My objective with this guide is to share this knowledge and information with a larger audience.

Why did I decide to write a guide dedicated to exercise for osteoporosis? It all started when a number of my clients at my Physiotherapy clinic had friends and family in need of an exercise program for osteoporosis but, because the friend or family member lived too far away for me to consult with in-person, my clients asked me if there were any exercise programs that I could recommend that were available online or in print. I searched online and reviewed different books and publications for exercise programs that I thought would be appropriate to recommend.

I was unable to find anything I felt was comprehensive enough to recommend to anyone interested in an exercise program for osteoporosis. The exercise programs that were available online or in print were limited in scope ("do weight bearing exercises to build bone"), did not take into account the individual's activity level and fracture risk, or were (in some cases) not based on scientific evidence.

I believe that an exercise program for the prevention and management of osteoporosis cannot take a "one-size-fits-all" approach, must cover a wide range of exercise activities that address balance, strength and flexibility, and must be supported by scientific evidence. The program must be designed to provide enough stress on the skeletal structure to encourage bone strengthening as well as allow you to develop the balance and strength required to reduce the chance of a fall. At the same time, there had to be a way to easily allow you to determine what program would be most appropriate for you based on your medical and activity profile. Finally, I felt that the program had to continually challenge you and keep you engaged – and be fun!

FOUR PRINCIPLES

As we age, our bone density decreases – potentially leading to osteoporosis. In fact, our bone density peaks at around the age of 30. The rate of decline depends on a number of factors and generally women experience a more dramatic decline than

> "The single thing that comes close to a magic bullet ... is exercise."
> - Dr. Frank Hu
> Epidemiologist
> Harvard School of Public Health

men. Fortunately, an exercise program designed to strengthen your bones can play a key role in slowing that rate of decline.

Studies show that regular weight bearing exercise and strength training can increase bone density in older adults by at least 1% per year. This may not sound like a lot, but it is significant considering that without the appropriate exercise, you could lose 1% or more bone density per year.

According to Dr. Frank Hu, epidemiologist at the Harvard School of Public Health: "The single thing that comes close to a magic bullet, in terms of its strong and universal benefits, is exercise."

The Exercise for Better Bones program is based on the following four principles:

» **Bone Building is Site Specific:** The effect of exercise on bone is specific to the location of the stresses caused by exercise[3]. If you want stronger leg bones, then brisk walking, squats, and lunges will help. But if you want stronger arm bones you have to use the bones and muscles in your arms by performing arm-specific exercises such as push-ups or bicep curls. Studies have shown that bones in the right arm of a right-handed tennis player have a greater density than bones in the left arm of the same player[4]. This means that if you want to be stronger throughout your body, you should have an exercise program that targets as many muscles and bones as possible. This is a special feature of this program. You get a progressive strength-training program that covers fourteen different exercises – that gradually builds over twelve weeks. The exercises have been chosen to specifically target the areas most commonly affected by low bone density.

» **High Mechanical Strains Affect Bone Health:** The loads or stresses placed on your bones during exercise need to be great enough to stimulate them[5,6]. If you can perform 15 repetitions of an exercise, you are not stressing the muscle enough to encourage bone building. (Although this is a good level when starting out and preparing your body to lift heavier weights.) When muscles contract strongly, the pulling effect stimulates your bones to respond and get stronger. The resistance/weight should challenge you enough that you can only repeat the exercise 8 to 12 times.

» **Weight Bearing Exercises are More Important Than Non-Weight Bearing Exercises:** Research has shown that weight bearing exercises are more effective than non-weight bearing exercises for improving bone density[7,8]. Any exercise where you bear weight through your skeleton is considered a weight bearing exercise. For example, brisk walking would be considered weight bearing for your hips whereas swimming and cycling are considered non-weight bearing for your hips.

» **Keep Your Bones on Their Toes:** Research in the area of bone building indicates that bones respond best to different stresses and new challenges[9]. This means that once you have mastered exercises at one level, you should progress to the next level. As such, I suggest that you try different cardiovascular/weight-bearing exercises. This will not only keep your program interesting and fun, but it will also keep your bones stimulated. In Chapter 8 of this guide, Cardiovascular Exercises, I provide a variety of activities by fracture risk level.

THE EXERCISE PROGRAMS

I am the author of the exercise programs in this guide. I am a Physical Therapist (licensed in California and registered to practice in Ontario) and Certified Strength and Conditioning Specialist with over 30 years of experience helping clients achieve their health and fitness goals.

The exercise programs were developed using evidence-based guidelines on the most effective exercise programs and activities for people with, or at risk of, osteoporosis. You can find the complete list of research papers used in the development of the programs at the end of this guide.

The exercise program incorporates all of the major areas important to building stronger bones:

- Postural Exercises
- Strength Exercises
- Balance Exercises
- Cardiovascular Exercises
- Flexibility Exercises

The programs that have been developed for you recognize you as an individual. The program you are assigned is based on your level of fitness and bone health. I strongly encourage you to follow the exercise program specific to your profile. (In Chapter 2 of this guide, I describe in detail how to determine the program you should follow.)

You will also be shown exercises to avoid since many exercises can actually increase your fracture risk.

The three fracture risk categories are: **Low, Moderate, and High**[10] and the four exercise program levels are: **Beginner, Active, Athletic, and Elite.** The levels are progressive. You can start at Beginner Level and progress to Active, Athletic, and finally to Elite. This guide contains **all** of the exercise program levels.

GOOD LUCK WITH YOUR PROGRAM

Now, onto Chapter 2 – How to Use This Guide. It is important that you read this chapter. It will make your experience with your program that much better.

Good luck and good bone-building!

Margaret Martin

Physical Therapist, Certified Strength and Conditioning Specialist.

2. How To Use This Guide

There is a lot of material and information in this guide developed specifically to help you improve your bone health. The challenge with presenting so much information is to deliver it in a way so that the reader does not get lost. To avoid that unfortunate situation, this chapter has been designed to help you navigate through the information and get you started on your exercise program.

Read this chapter carefully. I will cover the following topics:

» The contents of each chapter in this guide.

» How to locate important resources (such as your Exercise Plan).

» How and where you can determine your Exercise Level.

I am sure that you are eager to start your exercise program right away. I applaud you for your enthusiasm! However, there are a number of important foundational concepts covered in the early chapters of this guide that you should review before you start your program. Let me summarize these chapters.

In Chapter 3 – Bone and Body Basics, I cover your bone structure and how common day-to-day activities and certain exercises can increase your risk of a fracture. It is important that you read this chapter so that you understand why fractures happen under different conditions and why certain movements are best avoided or modified.

In Chapter 4 – Exercise Safety Tips, I present a number of key exercise recommendations. I talk about how you should develop an athletic stance (the athletic stance is referred to frequently throughout your exercise program, so you should make sure you understand it), how you should breathe while you exercise, how to get up and down from the floor, and how to safely use a Physio (exercise) ball.

In Chapter 5 – Exercises to Avoid, I identify popular exercises that should **not** be part of your exercise regimen. I encourage you to read this chapter. I think you will be surprised!

YOUR EXERCISE FOUNDATION

After reading and completing the activities in chapters 3 through 5, you will be ready to start your Exercise for Better Bones Program. Chapters 6 through 8 are used by all Levels.

In Chapter 6 – Posture Building Exercises, I cover the exercises that will improve your posture. This is an important chapter, since having a good posture is the foundation to safe and efficient movement patterns.

In Chapter 7 – Flexibility Exercises, I present my recommended flexibility or stretching exercises that are safe and effective for all fracture risk levels. Your Flexibility component will ensure that you stay limber. You should go through the flexibility exercises and see which ones challenge you. You may be very flexible in your upper body and yet tight in your legs, or vice versa. Focus on the areas that feel the tightest and try to increase your flexibility in those areas. Record which stretches you have done to ensure that you review them all periodically.

In Chapter 8 – Cardiovascular Exercises, I cover the appropriate and safe cardiovascular/ weight-bearing exercise activities for each fracture risk level. The Cardio/Weight Bearing exercises will provide you with the opportunity to work on your heart, as well as your bones and muscles. Don't forget to record your workout to ensure you are incorporating maximum bone building activities into each week.

MELIOGUIDE EXERCISE LEVELS

Chapters 9 through to 16 cover the Strength and Balance Exercises for each of the Exercise Levels:

» **Beginner** Strength Exercises (Chapter 9).

» **Beginner** Balance Exercises (Chapter 10).

» **Active** Strength Exercises (Chapter 11).

» **Active** Balance Exercises (Chapter 12).

» **Athletic** Strength Exercises (Chapter 13).

» **Athletic** Balance Exercises (Chapter 14).

» **Elite** Strength Exercises (Chapter 15).

» **Elite** Balance Exercises (Chapter 16).

DETERMINING YOUR EXERCISE PROGRAM LEVEL

Check the box that most closely describes your activity level:

☐ Have not exercised in months, years, or ever other than light housekeeping or gardening. **Level: Beginner.**

☐ Exercise once or twice weekly for over the past six months including using some light weights. Do all your own housework and yard work. **Level: Active.**

☐ Exercise three to four times weekly including using weights. Have used or are not intimidated by using the Physio (exercise) ball. Involved in light sports such as golfing, bowling, curling, or swimming. **Level: Athletic.**

☐ Exercise four to seven times weekly including using weights and a Physio (exercise) ball. Involved in higher-level sports such as hockey, soccer, or physique training. **Level: Elite.**

DETERMINING YOUR FRACTURE RISK LEVEL

Knowing your fracture risk will allow you to ensure you choose the most appropriate cardio/weight bearing exercises that stimulate bone without increasing your risk of a fracture.

The best way to determine your fracture risk is to follow guidelines established in FRAX – an online fracture risk assessment tool developed by the World Health Organization. If your Physician did not do your FRAX, I encourage you to visit **www.melioguide.com/frax** and review how to best answer the FRAX questions.

Finally, if your fracture risk is high (according to the FRAX guidelines), then I recommend that you omit the jumping and hopping exercises found in the Balance and Strength exercise sections in the Athletic and Elite levels.

WHERE TO FIND YOUR EXERCISE PLAN

Once you have determined your exercise level, visit **www.melioguide.com/exercise-plans**, find your program level, and download the PDF of your Exercise Plan.

I provide a 3-times-per-week exercise plan and a 6-times-per-week plan for you. When I present the option of working out 3-times-per-week or 6-times-per-week to my clients, most of them choose to work out 3-times-per-week.

Like many busy people these days, many of my clients find it hard to find the time to consistently complete their exercise programs and the 3-times-per-week commitment appears less onerous than the 6-times-per-week commitment.

However, when I explain to them that the 3-times-per-week plan means that they will have more exercises to complete in one session, some of them reconsider their original choice and opt for the 6-times-per-week plan.

The 6-times-per-week exercise plan will allow you to do fewer exercises per session while still getting one day off per week. By selecting the 6-times-per-week option, you spread your program over the week and reduce the amount of time per session.

No matter which of the two you choose, you will still be able to build your program over the 12-week time frame.

PROGRAM COMPONENTS

The **Postural Exercises** target muscles that need to be either stretched or strengthened to keep you in your best alignment.

The **Strength Exercises** should be followed as described in your Exercise Plan for your level. The strength training exercises require dumbbells and a burst-resistant Physio exercise ball. If you feel any discomfort with any of the strength exercises, you should consult with a qualified health professional, such as a Physical Therapist, before proceeding further.

The **Balance Exercises** will make you more stable and will have a direct impact on reducing your fracture risk. With practice, your balance will improve. Follow these instructions when you are performing your balance training:

» Choose among the exercises listed that challenge you.

» Make sure that you can hold your position for at least 10 seconds.

» Mix up the exercises from week to week for variety.

» Do a minimum of five minutes of balance training each session.

» Keep safety in mind by practicing your balance exercises in a safe location, such as a corner of a room with a sturdy chair in front of you for support.

The **Cardiovascular Exercise** section provides recommendations based on your fracture risk level along with suggestions that maximize weight bearing to benefit your bones.

The **Flexibility Exercises** are key to staying supple. As you strengthen your muscles, you also want to keep them flexible so that you optimize your posture and move with safe body mechanics.

STRENGTH TRAINING TIPS

I suggest you start in the following order for the **Strength Exercises** at your level:

» Get comfortable with your warm-up exercises; focus on your breathing and tummy tuck. Review all your exercise safety tips. Depending on how familiar you are with exercise training, you may want to gradually build over 12 weeks.

» If you are new to weight/resistance training, start with lighter weights, which allow you to fatigue by the fifteenth repetition. This will allow you to build the foundational components of your cells (mitochondria and microcapillaries).

» As the weeks progress you can gradually increase the resistance. Your goal should be to increase your weight or resistance to the point where your maximum number of reps before you fatigue is ten repetitions.

» If you have been weight or resistance training for at least three months, you should progress to the recommended intensity for bone building, which is a weight or resistance that allows you to fatigue by the tenth repetition.

» Once you are comfortable with the exercises and have started doing one set, I encourage you to add a second set. If time allows, you can even add a third set.

» You should never strength train the same muscle two days in a row. It is during your rest time that your body recovers from exercising and you get stronger.

EQUIPMENT NEEDS

You will not need to join a fitness center or a gym to complete your Exercise for Better Bones exercise program. If you do decide to use equipment located at one of these facilities, make sure you follow the guidelines below when choosing the equipment for you. The equipment that is required to allow you to complete the exercises in the privacy of your home will cost you less than a membership at a gym. Quality, not quantity, is what matters.

The following are my recommendations regarding equipment choices for your exercise program. The equipment you will need can be found at most major fitness stores.

Burst-Resistant Physio Ball

It is extremely important that the ball you get specifies "burst-resistant". This will ensure your safety. A number of Physio (exercise) balls on the market are not burst-resistant standard and there is the risk that the ball could burst while you are using it.

The following sizing guidelines will help you to determine the ball size you will need.

Your Height	Recommended Ball Height
Under 5'	45 cm or 17.7 inches
5' to 5' 4"	55 cm or 21.7 inches
5' 5" to 5' 11"	65 cm or 25.6 inches
6' plus	75 cm or 29.5 inches

As a rule, when sitting on a ball with your knees bent and your feet directly under your knees, your thighs should be parallel to the floor. This is the ideal ball size for exercising.

Free Weights (Dumbbells)

You will likely need a range of dumbbells ranging from 2 pounds to 20 pounds (or more, depending on your strength). As well, you will also need a 5 pound ankle weight. I suggest that you start with light weights and, as you get stronger, purchase the weights that keep you challenged.

Non-Slip Mat

If you do not have carpeting, a yoga type mat works very well for floor exercises. For more padding you may want to invest in an Airex type mat (a little pricey but they are very comfortable and will last you a lifetime).

Loop Bands

An elastic TheraBand loop band is used in the Postural Exercises and the Athletic Program.

½ Foam Roller

The Athletic Program uses a ½ Foam Roller for balance training.

TheraBand

TheraBand bands are available in a wide range of resistance levels with the level indicated by color of the band. Yellow is the TheraBand band with least resistance and black has the greatest resistance. Most beginners will be challenged with Yellow or Red TheraBand bands. The resistance progression for TheraBand bands is as follows:

- Yellow
- Red
- Green
- Blue
- Black

Stretching Strap or Rope

A number of the exercises use a strap or rope. My favorite type of rope is the 10 foot long, ¾ inch diameter smooth rope you can find at a hardware store. Make sure the rope is soft and smooth since you will be handling the rope in your hands and it may rub against your body during the exercises. If you are under 5 feet 4 inches in height, a bathrobe belt or yoga strap will do the trick.

MEDICAL ADVISORY

Not all exercises or activities are suitable for everyone. If you have any medical issues that affect exercise such as diabetes, or cardiac or respiratory problems, then we strongly recommend that you consult with a licensed or certified health professional before engaging in an exercise program. If you feel discomfort or pain during the exercise, stop.

Always seek the advice of your Physician, Physiotherapist, Physical Therapist, or other qualified health provider with any questions you may have regarding a medical condition or with reference to any content found in this guide. Never disregard professional medical advice or delay in seeking it because of something you have read in this guide.

MelioGuide is not responsible for any health problems that may result from training programs, products, or events you learn about through MelioGuide. If you engage in any exercise program you receive through MelioGuide, you agree that you do so at your own risk and are voluntarily participating in these activities.

SIGN UP FOR MY NEWSLETTER

I publish an online newsletter and I would love to see you subscribe to it. It is delivered to your email inbox. The newsletter is informative and covers a wide range of health topics and tips – not just bone health!

Visit **www.melioguide.com/enews** and sign up. I do not SPAM or share my email list with other parties. You can unsubscribe from the email list at any time by clicking on the unsubscribe link inside any of the emails that I send to you.

3. Bone and Body Basics

Research has demonstrated that when individuals have poor bone strength movements, whether they are moves associated with exercise or household chores, that incorporate a forward "slouching" of your back, will, over time, lead to compression fractures of your spine[1,2].

When you slouch forward, the weight of your head and upper body is transferred to the front of your vertebral body instead of being evenly distributed through your entire vertebral body. This concentration of weight on the front of your vertebral body can cause little fractures or micro fractures. With each micro fracture, your vertebral body weakens until eventually it collapses. The collapse of your vertebral body is known as a vertebral compression fracture.

Vertebral compression fractures can lead to a rounding of your upper back and a loss of height – making digesting food, eating, and breathing difficult. It also affects your balance and could lead to an increased risk of falling[3].

Vertebral compression fractures are the most common type of all osteoporotic fractures[4]. They often go undetected because the back pain associated with them may eventually diminish. Unfortunately, what most people do not realize is that once they have one compression fracture, their risk of another goes up significantly[5] unless they learn to move and exercise in a manner that supports their spine[6]. Unless intervention occurs with the right type of exercises, an individual who has experienced one vertebral compression fracture will be at significant risk for more vertebral fractures.

I encourage you to download my e-book at **www.melioguide.com/move-safe** that describes how to modify your daily activities to make them safer for your spine. It is filled with over forty practical examples that will save your spine.

In the next section, I describe your vertebral structure and why fractures occur.

The Vertebral Structure

The human spine is an incredible pillar made up of vertebrae – all held together by discs, ligaments, and muscles.

There are twenty-four vertebrae in the spine. Most people have seven vertebrae in their neck known as cervical vertebrae, twelve vertebra in their mid-torso known as thoracic vertebrae, and five vertebra in the low back known as lumbar vertebrae.

Figure 1, to the right, identifies the location of the different vertebrae in the spine.

The vertebral body is the weight-bearing part of your vertebrae. It is composed of two types of bone tissue: cortical and cancellous. Cortical bone is rigid and forms the hard outer layer of your vertebral body. Cancellous bone fills the inner cavity of your vertebral body and is porous in nature.

Cancellous bone is also referred to as trabecular or spongy bone. The inside of the cortical bone is supported by trabecula – the scaffolding structure within the cortical bone. The space between individual trabecula is the storage house for red and yellow marrow.

The thoracic vertebrae (located in the middle of the back) have the highest proportion of cancellous bone.

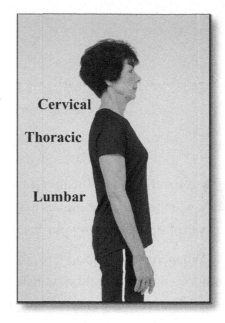

Figure 1

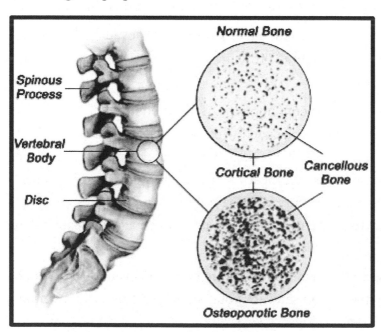

Figure 2

Figure 2, left, illustrates how the cortical and cancellous components make up a vertebral body.

In the upper magnified view, the cancellous bone tissue in the normal bone (represented by the light or white color) is quite dense and is able to provide support for the vertebral body.

(Note that the absence of bone tissue in the two circles is represented by the dark or black regions, while the presence of bone tissue is represented by the light or white areas.)

In the lower magnified view of the osteoporotic bone, the cancellous bone tissue is more porous. Individual trabecula have become thinner and, in some cases, have disappeared altogether.

The risk of fracture for the osteoporotic vertebra, in the lower part of Figure 2, has increased (as compared to the vertebral body of the normal bone) because it has a lower number of cross-linking trabecula and a thinner honeycomb structure.

Our bone density peaks when we reach around 30 years of age. After that, our bone density starts to decrease. As bone density within the skeleton is lost, it is lost at a faster rate in cancellous bone. As a result, the vertebral body – composed largely of cancellous bone – is at an elevated risk of fracturing.

Recommendations

There are a number of things that you can do to reduce your risk of fracture in this part of your body:

»   Follow the exercise program in this guide. It will allow you to build your bones, cardiovascular strength, and flexibility, and reduce your risk of falls without practicing exercises that increase the risk of a fracture.

»   Practice the posture building exercises in Chapter 6 to improve your posture. Performing activities with a good posture decreases your risk of a spinal fracture.

»   I encourage you to download my e-book at **www.melioguide.com/move-safe** and learn how you should modify your daily activities. To function day-to-day, we need to bend forward. We need to pick up items from the floor, load the dishwasher, etc. I am not advocating that you no longer do these activities. I suggest you learn to move with good body mechanics. The bending forward motion should occur from the hip and knees and not your spine.

»   Certain exercises, including some Yoga and Pilates[7] poses, can cause strain on the vertebrae of a person with low bone density or osteoporosis and will increase your risk of vertebral fracture. If you are a Yoga practitioner or instructor you should read my book, *Yoga for Better Bones*. Yoga for Better Bones outlines the modifications that can be made to specific Yoga poses to ensure that they do not increase your risk of fracture.

4. Exercise Safety Tips

When I start working with a new client, I always devote time (before they start their exercise program) teaching them how to breath efficiently, how to safely get up and down from the floor, and how to activate their deep abdominal muscles. This chapter will cover these and other very important safety basics.

The exercise safety tips in this chapter should be carefully reviewed and followed by anyone who has low bone density, osteopenia, or osteoporosis. When you practice these safe exercise habits on a regular basis and incorporate them into your exercise program, you will find that many of the habits will become part of your daily routine.

Maintaining an athletic stance when doing housework, breathing properly when you are playing with the kids, and keeping your tummy tucked (while doing activities that involve pushing, pulling, and carrying) will make each of these activities safer for your spine. Over time and with practice, your new good form will extend from your exercise program into all your daily activities.

This exercise program has been designed to minimize the risk of fracture during the prescribed exercise activity.

I recommend that you read this chapter carefully and review it periodically to ensure that you are following proper form.

USE YOUR BREATH TO SUPPORT YOU

If you watch a baby sleep you will see the rise and fall of their tummy. You will not see the upper chest move. The main muscle of respiration we are born to breathe with is the diaphragm. The fibers of the diaphragm originate from our lower ribs and attach to the vertebral bodies of our lumbar spine.

When you inhale fully from your diaphragm, your lower ribs expand along with your upper abdominal area and as you exhale your lower ribs and upper abdominal area release. When we are anxious, nervous, or stressed breathing patterns often become shallow. Stress tells our body to fight or get ready to run. Under stress, we start to breathe with our upper chest, neck, and shoulder muscles.

Taking time before meals, sleeping, and exercise can help you focus on natural breathing, program your breathing pattern, and relieve tension in your shoulders and neck.

How will correct breathing make me stronger?

Your diaphragm is your largest respiratory muscle. It divides the space between you thoracic cavity and your abdominal cavity. It makes up the superior portion of your inner core. Aside from getting more oxygen to your working muscles, when you use your diaphragm correctly, you are complementing the team of muscles that keeps your spine stable, assisting in your overall stability.

How are breathing and exercise related?

Breathing is an integral component of an exercise program. In order to achieve the full benefit from an exercise program your breathing needs to be rhythmic and full.

How will I know if I am breathing with my diaphragm?

Follow these steps to determine whether you're using your diaphragm to breathe:

» Begin by breathing in through your nose and out through pursed lips, as though gently blowing through a straw.

» Place one hand to rest gently on the area of your abdomen just below your rib cage and above your belly button. You should feel your hand rise with each inhalation and fall with each exhalation.

» Next, place your hands to rest gently onto your lower ribs. You should feel your hands rise, as your ribs expand with each inhalation and fall with each exhalation.

As mentioned earlier, your diaphragm makes up the top portion of your inner core. What we have not yet mentioned is the lower portion of your inner core – your pelvic floor. The rhythm of your pelvic floor follows the rhythm of your diaphragm. As you inhale your pelvic floor relaxes

Exercise Safety Tips

and as you exhale it gently tightens. Like the rhythm of the diaphragm, the rhythm of the pelvic floor is often lost with life's challenges. The next section is there to help you regain the rhythm.

TIGHTEN YOUR LOWER TUMMY

Throughout your exercise program, reminders are written into each strength building exercise to "tighten your lower tummy as you exhale." The following will guide you through this step:

» Begin by breathing in with a full relaxed breath through your nose and out through pursed lips, as though gently blowing through a straw.

Your abdominal muscles and pelvic floor muscles are meant to work together. It is best to use muscles of the pelvic floor to enhance the muscle action of the deep abdominals. For women, this would be equivalent of gently squeezing a tampon. For men, imagine walking into cold water. Your scrotum and penis gently retract into your body. Another analogy that has been shown to awaken your deep abdominals is to imagine pulling your front pelvic bones towards one another as you exhale. Please do not do a pelvic tilt. I want you to learn to use your deep muscles with your spine in a neutral position.

KEEP YOUR TONGUE ON THE ROOF OF YOUR MOUTH

When you perform any of the upper body strengthening exercises or ball exercises, you should keep your tongue to the roof of your mouth. This encourages the deep stabilizing muscles of your neck to support you during the exercise.

DEVELOP AN ATHLETIC STANCE

It is important that you develop a stance when you exercise that provides optimum support and balance. This is commonly known as an "athletic stance." When you are in an athletic stance, your weight is distributed evenly, you have good balance and stability, and you are able to confidently perform an activity. Follow these instructions to develop an athletic stance:

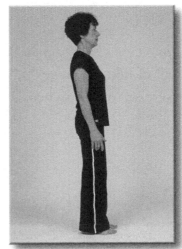

» Stand with your weight evenly distributed between both feet

» Evenly distribute your weight between the base of your big toe, little toe and the center of your heel

» Soften your knees, gently tighten the muscles of your upper thighs

» Lengthen the space between your rib cage and pelvis

» Gently bring your shoulder blades towards one another and down

» Draw the crown of your head to the sky

Exercise Safety Tips

GETTING UP AND DOWN FROM FLOOR – OPTION 1

Some of the exercises in your exercise program may require that you lie on the floor either on your tummy (face down) or on your back. It is important that you learn how to safely lower yourself to the floor to perform your exercise. You will also need to know how to safely get up from the floor. I will cover both getting up and down.

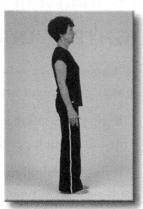

The following are the individual steps for getting safely onto your tummy starting from a standing position:

» From your standing position, slowly step back and slowly lower yourself onto one knee. Support yourself with a chair if you need.

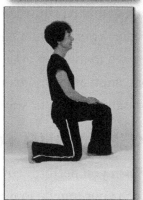

» Continue to carefully lower yourself to the crawl position on all fours.

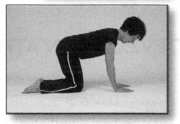

» Crawl forward on your hands or forearms until you are face down and flat on the floor.

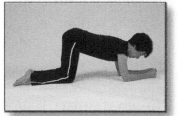

To safely get back up into a standing position, simply reverse the order of the steps described above until you are in a standing position.

Practicing getting up and down from the floor removes much of the fear of falling. However, if it is too strenuous you can do the floor exercises on a firm bed.

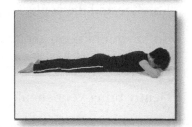

Exercise Safety Tips

GETTING UP AND DOWN FROM FLOOR – OPTION 2

MOVEMENT

» From your hands and knees you can lower yourself to sit on the outside of your thigh.

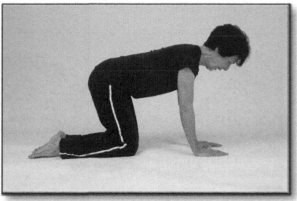

» Lower yourself to your side.

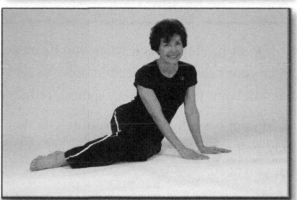

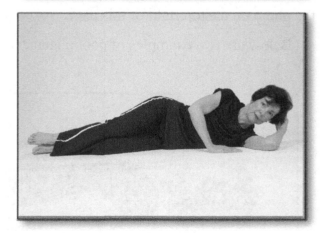

» Roll over onto your back or front (not shown in photos).

To safely get back up into a standing position, simply reverse the order of the steps described above until you are in a standing position.

Exercise Safety Tips

HEAD POSITION

Keep your head in a neutral alignment position (or as close as you can) throughout your exercises. This position is demonstrated in the next two photos.

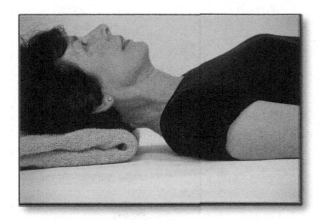 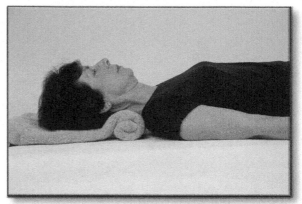

If your head tilts back when you lie on your back, you should place as many towel layers under your head as you need in order to get your eyes pointing to the ceiling. This is one area you will want your therapist, spouse, or friend to guide you.

In your best alignment position, you should be able to comfortably swallow. With time, your body will regain some of its lost range and you will be able to reduce the layers of towel support that you need.

For additional neck support, you may choose to roll the towel under your neck as shown in the photo on the top right of this page.

Below are two examples of poor alignment.

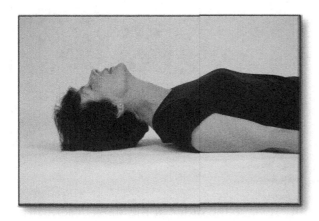 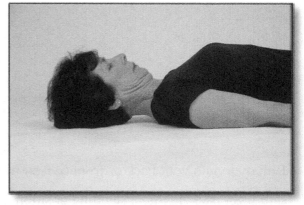

Exercise Safety Tips

SAFELY USING A PHYSIO BALL

If you have not used a Physio Ball before (or even if you are a veteran), I recommend that you create a small "fence" around you so that the ball will not move far in case you roll unexpectedly. A set of cushions from your couch is ideal.

Here are some important tips on the safe use of a Physio Ball.

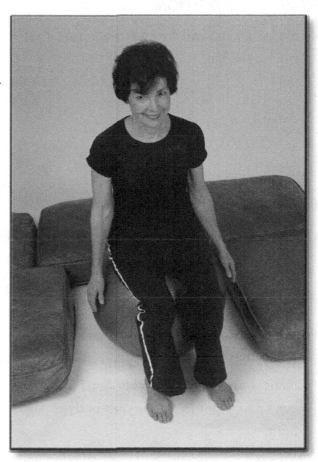

» Use extra caution by placing your sofa cushions on either side, behind, or in front of you depending on the exercise.

» You want to allow yourself an inch or so of "play." This will give you the dynamic benefit of the ball without the risk of injuring yourself should you lose your balance.

» Another option when getting on and off the ball into a table top position is to create a valley between your sofa and your sofa cushions.

Exercise Safety Tips

GETTING ON THE PHYSIO BALL SAFELY

A number of the exercises in the Athletic and Elite exercise programs require the use of a Physio Ball. It is important that you learn how to get on a Physio Ball without bending forward from your spine.

STARTING POSITION:

» Sit tall on the ball with your hands resting on either side of the ball.

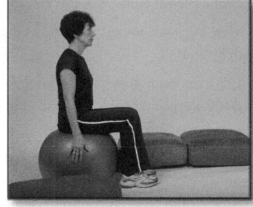

MOVEMENT:

» Keep your feet near to you, your knees should be at almost a right angle through the walk out.

» Slowly walk your feet out in front of you as you lower you buttocks and allow your lower back to rest against the ball.

» When you feel the ball resting under your shoulder blades, start by raising your hips, then lower your head and shoulders until your body is parallel to the floor.

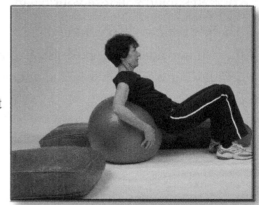

» You should have the ball under the top half of your shoulder blades with your head resting fully on the ball but without feeling like you are holding yourself up with your neck. This position, when done properly, will provide maximum comfort and create minimal strain during your Athletic and Elite ball exercises.

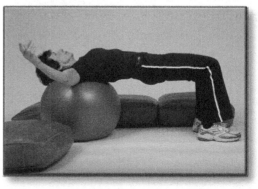

To return to the original upright position:

» Drop your buttocks.

» Keep your chin tucked as you walk back up to a seated position placing your hands on the ball for support.

Exercise Safety Tips

POSITIONING YOUR LEGS FOR FLOOR EXERCISES

The correct position of your legs is sometimes referred to as the "effortless resting position."

You want to place your feet just the right distance from your buttocks so that your legs rest easily. Your feet and knees should be hip width apart.

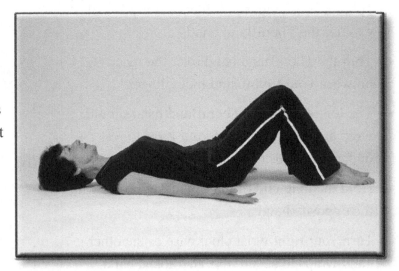

HOW TO REDUCE THE STRAIN ON YOUR SHOULDERS

Some of the exercises (depending on your level) require you to hold your weight through your arms. This can cause strain on your shoulders if the exercise is not executed properly. An example is the Push Up.

As you start this type of exercise you should set your shoulders by gently drawing your shoulder blades downward and inward toward each other.

Exercise Safety Tips

WRAPPING THE THERABAND BAND

The photos to the right provide a description of how to use the TheraBand band.

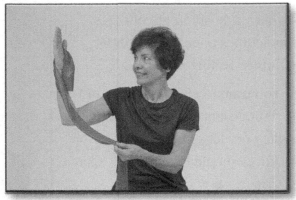

» Trail the TheraBand band over the space between your thumb and index finger.

» The long end of the TheraBand band should wrap around the back of your hand to rest under your fifth finger.

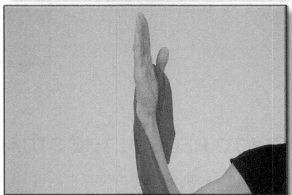

» Hold the long end of the TheraBand band with the opposite hand.

» Turn your right wrist clockwise as the other hand wraps to secure the Theraband band.

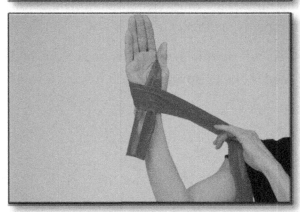

» If you need to increase the resistance of the band make additional turns of your wrists.

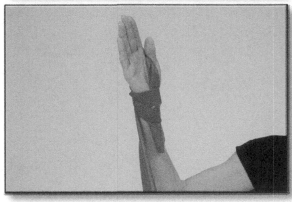

Exercise Safety Tips

5. Exercises to Avoid

The next time you go to the bookstore, visit the area in the store where they have the fitness magazines. Find a magazine with a "hard body" on the cover – you know what I mean. Read one of the many articles that promises to make you look like the model on the cover. Take note of the exercises they recommend that involve crunches – and avoid them!

Research and clinical studies have shown that flexion of the osteoporotic spine, especially in situations where force is applied, can lead to fractures of the vertebrae. Unfortunately, this scientific fact is not well known within the fitness community and, as a result, you will find many Personal Trainers (and some medical professionals!) in books and magazines encouraging exercises (like traditional crunches) that cause flexion and potentially put you at risk of a fracture.

I frequently have clients with known diagnosis of osteoporosis come to my clinic for a bone-friendly exercise program once they realize that the Personal Trainer they have been using at a gym has not taken into consideration their specific health needs when assigning them an exercise program. They are surprised (and frequently shocked) when they learn that the exercises that they have been doing, under the guidance of a Personal Trainer, have actually been *increasing* their risk of a fracture.

If you remember from Chapter 3, Body and Bone Basics, flexion and the combinations of flexion and rotation are not recommended for people with osteopenia or osteoporosis. Many of the exercises to avoid, covered in this chapter, encourage either flexion or rotation (or both).

Many of these exercises have been with us for years. You have probably done a number of them in your past (hopefully for the last time!). You may be surprised by some of the exercises I am asking you not to do. Let's start with the most popular of exercises: the traditional crunch or sit-up – used by many people to build their abs.

CRUNCHES

Traditional "crunches" (also known as sit-ups) are popular with most exercise programs for development and strengthening of the abdominal muscles. There are many variations of the crunch. The illustrations to the right demonstrate two of the many variations.

Due to the risk associated with vertebral fractures, this exercise is not advised for people with low bone density or osteoporosis.

There are many other exercises you can do to strengthen your abdominal muscles that are safe and do not place your spine at risk. These are covered in the Strength Exercises section in each of the exercise program Levels.

You can also refer to my book, ***Strengthen Your Core***, available in both Kindle and print formats, for a complete and safe program to strengthen your core.

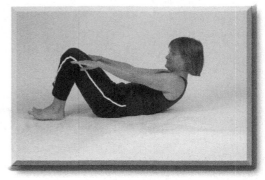

Unsafe

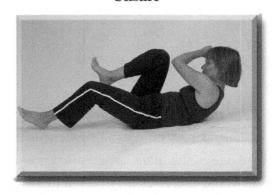

Unsafe

CHEST FLY

When using gym equipment, most women have to adjust their body position to accommodate the machines. The Chest Fly machine may cause undue stress on the vertebrae, possibly risking a fracture for people diagnosed with osteoporosis. I recommend you approach this exercise with caution.

CHEST PRESS

When using gym equipment, this exercise (like its sister exercise, the Chest Fly) causes undue stress on the vertebrae, possibly risking a fracture for people with low bone density or osteoporosis. I recommend that you avoid this exercise and that you avoid using this piece of gym equipment altogether unless you can keep your spine in perfect alignment.

Unsafe

Exercises to Avoid

KNEE EXTENSIONS

This exercise encourages a "slouched" posture, potentially risking a fracture of the vertebrae for people with osteoporosis.

If you are able to perform this exercise without the forward lean (the slouch position), then you should be okay with the exercise. In my experience, most individuals find it difficult to maintain their posture while repeatedly doing this exercise and over time, they gravitate back to the slouch position.

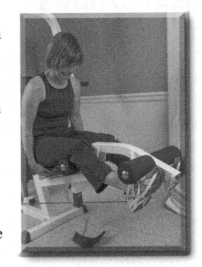

Unsafe

LAT PULL DOWN (BEHIND THE HEAD)

Doing a lat pull down behind your head, as illustrated in the photo on the right, places excess stress on your shoulders, neck, and spine. I strongly advise that you do not do this exercise this way.

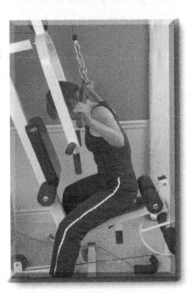

Unsafe

A lat pull down, when done correctly, as illustrated in the photo to the immediate right, is an excellent exercise. The following are some simple instructions to follow for good "lat pull down" form:

» The bar should be pulled down in front of you, just below your chin.

» You should keep your breastbone high and tuck your shoulder blades towards your pockets on the back of your pants as your elbows descend.

Safe

Exercises to Avoid

SEATED ROWS

This exercise, when done incorrectly, encourages a "slouched" posture, potentially risking a fracture to the vertebrae for people with osteoporosis. This slouch position is illustrated in the photo to the immediate right. Note the curvature of the upper back caused by the model leaning forward to follow the cord. This position should to be avoided.

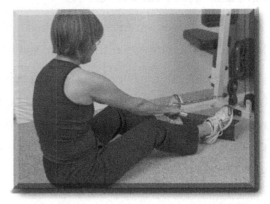

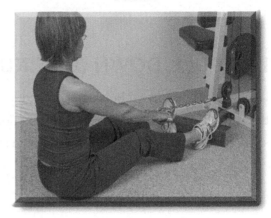

Unsafe

This exercise can be performed safely when the person assumes a better posture – as illustrated in the picture to the immediate right. Note that the model has kept her posture straight and aligned. There is no forward lean or slouch.

The challenge for most people will be to maintain a straight posture when they pull, pick up, and return the pulley to the rack. If you decide that this an exercise you want to keep in your routine, make sure that you maintain your posture throughout the execution of this exercise.

Safe

TOE TOUCH WITH A TWIST

The toe touch with a twist is often the staple flexibility exercise in many Personal Training routines. The problem with this exercise is that it encourages a twist and bend in the spine, potentially risking a fracture to the vertebrae for people with osteoporosis.

This exercise is high up on the list of exercises to avoid because it combines both flexion and rotation. There is no way to modify the exercise to make it safe for you. This one is best avoided altogether.

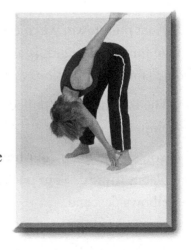

Unsafe

Exercises to Avoid

HAMSTRING STRETCHES

This stretch (and its variations) encourages flexion, potentially risking vertebral fracture for people diagnosed with osteoporosis.

The three photos illustrate common variations of this exercise.

The traditional hamstring stretch is frequently used to increase flexibility. Note that in the demonstrations, the model has a curvature of the back caused by the forward lean. This curvature or flexion needs to be avoided by people with low bone density and osteoporosis.

In our Flexibility section, there are excellent and very effective hamstring stretches that do not put your spine at risk. I suggest you avoid the traditional hamstring stretch demonstrated on this page and instead use the exercises in the Flexibility section of the Exercise for Better Bones program.

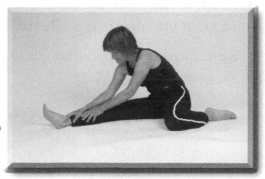

Unsafe

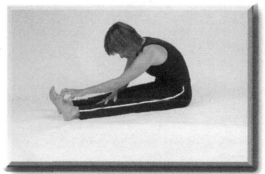

Unsafe

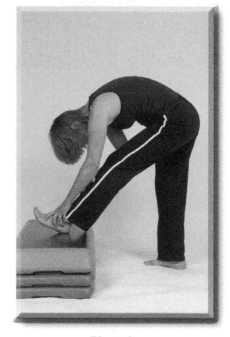

Unsafe

Exercises to Avoid

BACK STRETCHES

This back stretch exercise position, illustrated in the photo below, encourages flexion of the spine with a lot of loading – potentially risking vertebrae fracture for people with osteoporosis.

Since there are no modifications that can be made to this exercise to address its shortcomings, the exercise is best avoided.

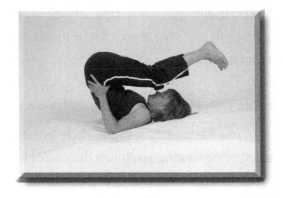

Unsafe

Exercises to Avoid

48

CARDIOVASCULAR EXERCISE CONSIDERATIONS

Good posture is important to maintain throughout your cardio routine. Make sure that you maintain proper posture and avoid positions that cause flexion of the spine.

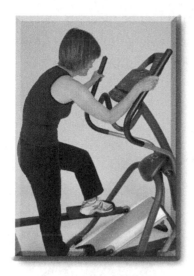

Unsafe

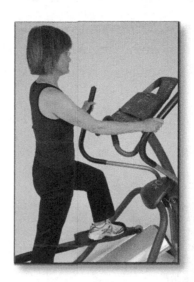

Safe

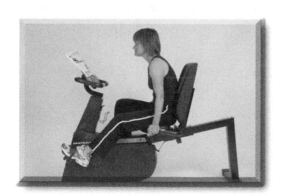

Unsafe

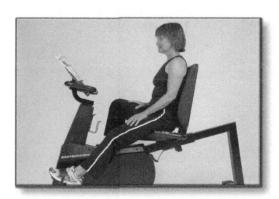

Safe

Exercises to Avoid

YOGA FOR BETTER BONES

Certain exercises, including some Yoga and Pilates poses, can cause strain on the vertebrae of a person with low bone density or osteoporosis and will increase your risk of vertebral fracture. If you are a Yoga practitioner or instructor you should read my book, *Yoga for Better Bones.*

In *Yoga for Better Bones*, I outline the modifications that can be made to specific Yoga poses to ensure that they do not increase your risk of fracture. Below is a illustration from the book demonstrating a Yoga pose, Janu Sirsasana, that requires modification.

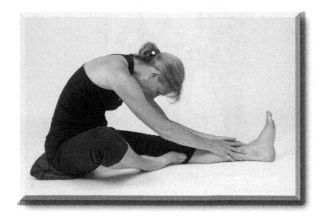

Unsafe

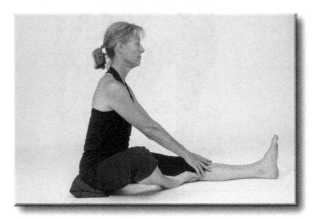

Safe

Exercise to Avoid

A SAFER EXERCISE PROGRAM

I am sure that you have done many of these exercises at one point in your life. It is now time to leave them behind and to move onto an exercise program that builds bone strength and reduces the risk of fracture in a safe and effective way. You should congratulate yourself for taking a step in the right direction. You are about to embark on your program!

Exercises to Avoid

6. Posture Building Exercises

Most of the activities of everyday life bring us into forward positions. If we are not meticulous about our posture throughout the day, then gravity will gradually pull our head forward and soon our spine will follow.

Flexion of your spine happens with a slouched posture. This flexion motion has been shown to increase your risk of a vertebral fracture. The purpose of this chapter is to lead you through a complete series of exercises to build your posture.

The purpose for all the postural exercises is to assist you in stretching and strengthening the muscles you need to regain better alignment. The main goal is to reduce your risk of a vertebral fracture.

Not everyone will have to complete the posture building exercises. If you are able to maintain a proper postural position, you can skip this chapter. Here is a Quick Posture Test for you to see if you would benefit from the exercises in this chapter.

A Quick Posture Test

» Stand tall against a wall with your heels 4 to 6 inches away from the base board.

» Bend your knees slightly. Keep your eyes horizontal. Measure how far the back of your head is from the wall.

If the back of your head is not comfortably resting on the wall then you would benefit from doing the postural exercises in this chapter.

Here are some guidelines to follow:

» Begin in the order they are presented, unless indicated otherwise by your health practitioner.

» On the first week, start with five to ten repetitions of the first three posture-stretching exercises and repeat the exercises every day. Hold each stretch for one to two seconds.

» On <u>week two</u> add the next four posture-stretching exercises, completing five to ten repetitions of each exercise every day. Hold each stretch for one to two seconds.

» On <u>week three</u> add the next three posture-strength exercises, completing five to ten repetitions of each exercise every other day. Hold each strength exercise for two to three seconds.

» On <u>week four</u> add the last three posture-strength exercises, completing five to ten repetitions of each exercise every other day. Hold each strength exercise for two to three seconds.

I encourage you to continue with these exercises until they can be done with ease and comfort. As you build your posture I encourage you to also work on your balance exercises.

With all postural stretches and strengthening exercises you should:

1. Keep your head and neck in optimal alignment.
2. Keep the small of your back a hands-width from the floor.

The average weight of the head is between 4.5 and 5.0 kilograms (between 10 and 11 pounds). You want the weight of your head to be bearing down through your spine and not falling in front of it!

The postural exercises outlined in this chapter are essential for anyone who has excessive thoracic kyphosis (a pronounced hump or rounding of the upper back) and is unable to hold their head in alignment over their body. Perfect posture is the foundation for all movements.

Please refer to the Head Position section in Chapter 4 – Exercise Tips and determine how many towel layers you will need for your postural exercises.

I have broken the postural building exercises into postural stretching exercises and postural strengthening exercises. You can tell which category each exercise belongs to by looking at the bottom corner of each page.

For each of the postural stretching exercises I have identified where you should feel the stretch. This is to help you to relax into the stretch knowing you are doing the correct movement.

For each of the postural strengthening exercises I have listed the prime or main muscles involved in executing the exercise as well as which part of your skeleton gets the most stimulation from the exercise.

CHIN TUCK STRETCH

WHERE YOU SHOULD FEEL IT:

» Base of your skull.

STARTING POSITION:

» Lie on your back, place your arms out from your side with palms up, your knees bent.

» Inhale using your diaphragm (your tummy should rise).

» This would be a good time to review "Head Position" in Chapter 4.

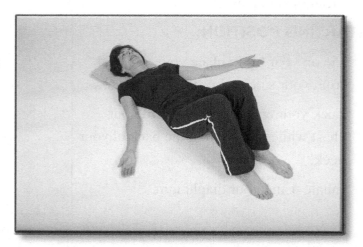

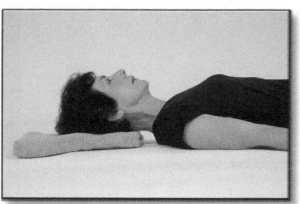

MOVEMENT:

Exhale and gently tighten your lower tummy as you:

» Tuck your chin slightly towards your chest while lengthening the back of your neck.

» Keep the small of your back a hand-width from the floor.

» Hold this position for 1 to 2 seconds and repeat 5 to 10 times.

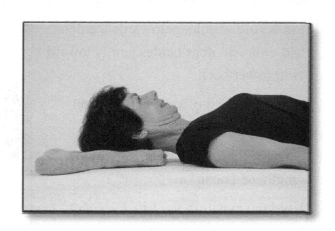

Postural Stretching Exercises

SHOULDER TUCK STRETCH

WHERE YOU SHOULD FEEL IT:

» Front of shoulder.

STARTING POSITION:

» Lie on your back, place your arms out from your side, palms up, knees bent.

» Tuck your chin slightly toward your chest while lengthening the back of your neck.

» Inhale using your diaphragm.

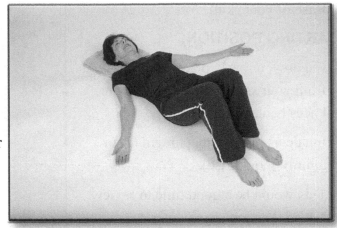

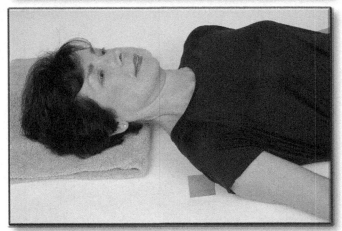

MOVEMENT:

Exhale and gently tighten your lower tummy as you:

» Press your shoulders towards the floor and your shoulder blades gently toward your lower back.

» Keep the small of your back a hand-width from the floor.

» Be mindful to keep your neck in the lengthened position.

» Hold this position for 1 to 2 seconds, relax, and repeat 5 times.

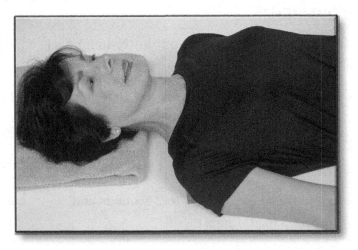

Postural Stretching Exercises

CHEST STRETCH – FLOOR

WHERE YOU SHOULD FEEL IT:

» Chest.

» Upper arms.

STARTING POSITION:

» Lie on your back with your hands resting over your ears, elbows pointing to the ceiling, and your knees bent.

» Inhale using your diaphragm.

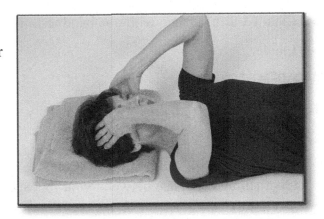

MOVEMENT:

Exhale and gently tighten your lower tummy as you:

» Press your elbows downward and outward into the floor.

» Keep the small of your back a hand-width from the floor.

» Hold for 1 to 2 seconds and repeat 5 times.

» Be mindful to keep your neck in the lengthened position.

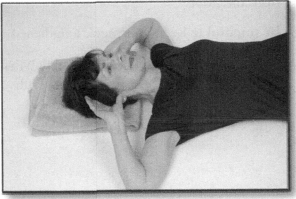

» If the backs of your arms do not touch the floor, you can place folded towels or pillows by your side so that you have something to push against. You should try to gradually reduce the support until you can get your arms to the floor.

TIP:

» This exercise can also be done standing up against a wall or sitting tall in a chair.

Postural Stretching Exercises

ARM REACH STRETCH

WHERE YOU SHOULD FEEL IT:

» Anywhere from your low back to your arm.

STARTING POSITION:

» Lie on a firm surface with one hand resting beside your ear (of the same side).

» Inhale.

MOVEMENT:

Exhale and gently tighten your lower tummy as you:

» Slide your hand along the floor reaching toward the wall behind you, gently lengthening the space between your rib cage and pelvis.

» Keep the small of your back a hand-width from the floor.

» Be mindful to keep your neck lengthened.

» Return your arm to the start position, repeat 5 times and then repeat the exercise with your other arm.

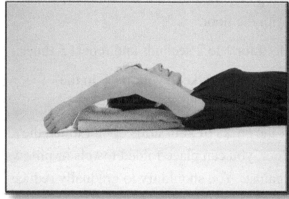

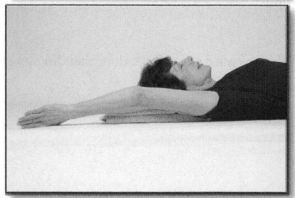

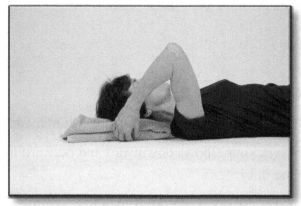

Postural Stretching Exercises

EAR TO CHEST STRETCH

WHERE YOU SHOULD FEEL IT:

» Upper back.

» Shoulders.

» Neck.

STARTING POSITION:

» Keep your back tall and turn your head to the left so that your chin lines up with your left breast.

» Inhale.

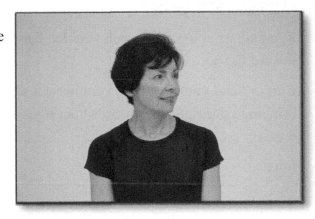

MOVEMENT:

Exhale as you:

» Curl or bend your neck one vertebra at a time bringing your right ear towards your right breast.

» At the end of the movement, bring your right hand to rest by your left ear to gently assist the stretch.

» Hold for 1 to 2 seconds and repeat 5 times.

» Return to start position and repeat on the other side.

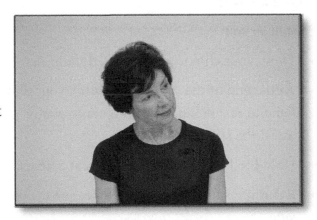

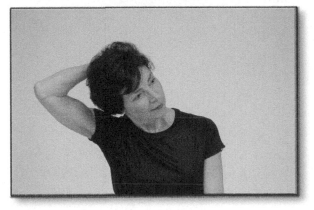

Postural Stretching Exercises

CHIN TO CHEST STRETCH

WHERE YOU SHOULD FEEL IT:

» Upper back.

» Shoulders.

» Neck.

STARTING POSITION:

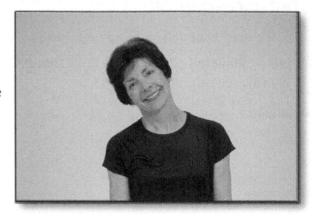

» Keep tall as you gently reach your left hand toward the floor.

» Curl or bend your neck one vertebra at a time bringing your right ear towards your right breast.

» Inhale.

MOVEMENT:

Exhale as you:

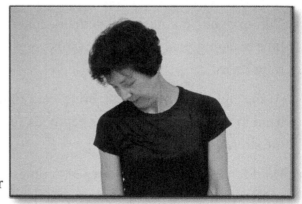

» Draw your chin towards your right breast.

» At the end of the movement, bring your right hand to rest behind your left ear to gently assist the stretch.

» Hold for 1 to 2 seconds and repeat 5 times.

» Return to start position and repeat on the other side.

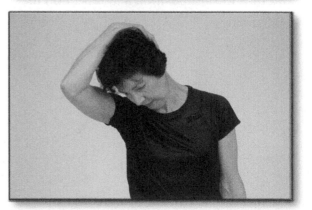

Postural Stretching Exercises

SPINAL STRETCH

WHERE YOU SHOULD FEEL IT:

» Abdominal muscles.

» Spine.

STARTING POSITION:

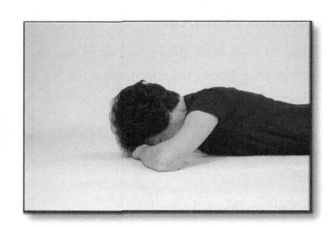

» Lie on your stomach, forehead resting on hands with elbows facing outward, palms down.

» Tuck your chin slightly.

» Inhale.

MOVEMENT:

Exhale and gently press the front of your pelvis into the floor as you:

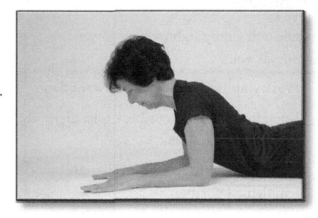

» Tuck both elbows into your side, coming to rest directly under your shoulders.

» Relax into the stretch as you try to get your breastbone parallel to the wall in front of you.

» Hold 1 to 2 seconds and return to your start position.

» Repeat 5 times.

TIP:

» Visualize your breast-bone parallel to the wall in front of you.

» If you find this stretch to be difficult or you feel discomfort in your low back, you should begin by using one to two pillows under your pelvis. As you regain your flexibility, you may reduce the size (and number) of the pillows until you can do this without any support from pillows.

» Keep your eyes fixed on your hands as you lift up.

Postural Stretching Exercises

NECK PRESS

TARGETS:

» Muscles: Erector spinae and semispinalis (the deep muscles in your neck).

» Bones: Spine.

STARTING POSITION:

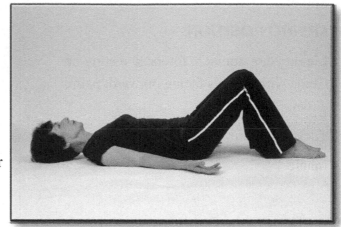

» Lie on your back, place your arms out from your sides, palms up and your knees bent.

» Tuck your chin slightly towards your chest while lengthening the back of your neck.

» Inhale using your diaphragm.

MOVEMENT:

Exhale and gently tighten your lower tummy as you:

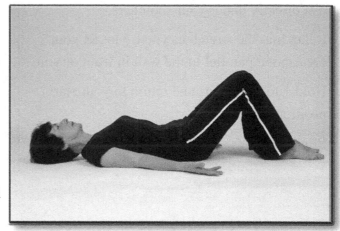

» Press your head downward toward floor.

» Keep the small of your back a hand-width from the floor.

» Be mindful to keep your neck in the lengthened position.

» Hold this position for 2 to 3 seconds and repeat 5 times.

TIP:

» Unlike the Chin Tuck Stretch, you should feel the muscles at the back of your neck tighten (or contract) rather than stretch.

» Remember to keep your head alignment as discussed in "Head Position" in Chapter 4.

Postural Strengthening Exercises

SHOULDER STABILIZATION

TARGETS:

» Muscles: Rotator cuff (back of shoulder blade), rhomboids (deep muscle of upper back).

» Bones: Spine.

STARTING POSITION:

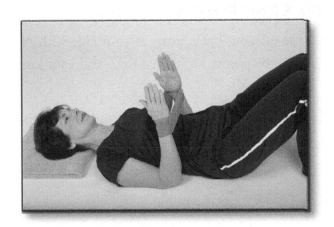

» On your back in your best alignment/sitting tall/standing tall.

» Loop a band, the width of your shoulders, around your wrists.

» Bend elbows at a right angle.

» Inhale.

MOVEMENT:

Exhale and gently tighten your lower tummy as you:

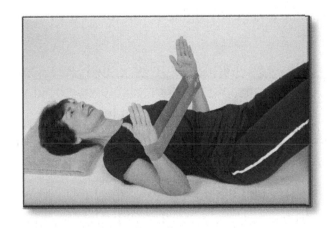

» Slide your shoulder blades downward and together.

» Draw your elbows into your side and press outwards through your wrist.

» Hold 2 to 3 seconds and repeat 5 times.

TIPS:

» There should be very little motion but maximum effort.

» If you do not have a loopband, then a belt, rope, or heavy TheraBand band will work.

» Think of your elbows as pivot points.

Postural Strengthening Exercises

OVERHEAD PRESS

TARGETS:

» Lower trapezius.

STARTING POSITION:

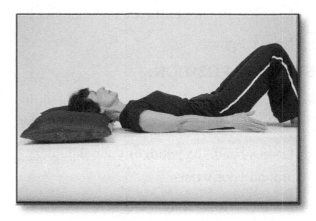

» Lie on your back, arms at your side with thumbs pointed to the ceiling, and your knees bent.

» Use as much support under your head as you did with the Neck Press exercise.

MOVEMENT:

Exhale and gently tighten your lower tummy as you:

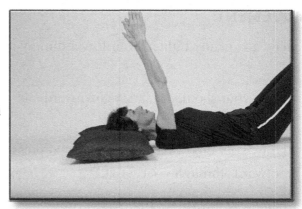

» Raise your arms overhead so that you press your arms into the floor next to your head with your elbows straight but not locked.

» If you do not reach the floor, push into a soft chair or pillows placed beside your head.

» Press into the floor/pillows for 2 to 3 seconds.

» Return your arms to the start position and then repeat 5 times.

TIPS:

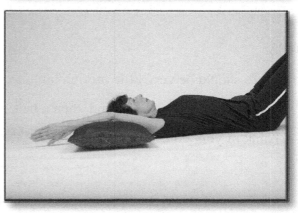

» Press using your upper arms and back.

» Avoid bending your elbows.

» Using your abdominals, keep the small of your back a hand-width from the floor and do not let your lower ribs lift off the floor.

» Be mindful to keep your neck in the lengthened position.

Postural Strengthening Exercises

NECK LIFT

TARGETS:

» Muscles: Erector spinae and semispinalis (the deep muscles in your neck).

» Bones: Spine.

STARTING POSITION:

» Lie face down on floor with legs straight.

» Rest forehead on rolled towel.

» Inhale using your diaphragm.

» Use as much support under your head as you did with the Neck Press exercise.

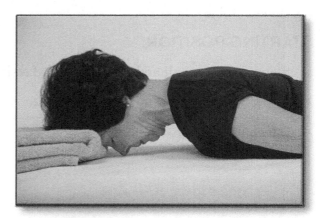

MOVEMENT:

Exhale and as you gently press the front of your pelvis into the floor:

» Raise the back of your head towards the ceiling.

» Keep your gaze at the towels.

» Hold 2 to 3 seconds and repeat 5 times

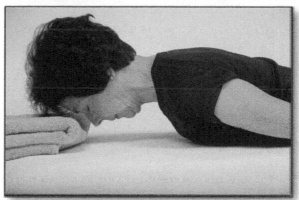

TIPS:

» Imagine that you are holding an orange under your chin throughout the movement.

» Large-breasted women will benefit from using a larger roll under their forehead, thereby bringing their head to a more neutral position.

Postural Strengthening Exercises

ARM PULL BACK

TARGETS:

» Muscles: Lower trapezius.

» Bones: Spine.

STARTING POSITION:

» Stand facing a wall and arms over head resting on the wall.

» Toes and your nose should be as close to wall as possible.

» Inhale using your diaphragm.

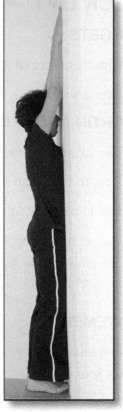

MOVEMENT:

Exhale and gently tighten your lower tummy as you:

» Slide your shoulder blade(s) down as you lift your arm(s) off the wall.

» Hold for 2 to 3 seconds and return to start position.

» Repeat 5 times.

» Repeat movement using other arm.

TIP:

» You may also lift off with both arms simultaneously, as shown here.

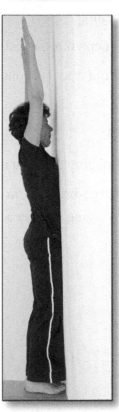

Postural Strengthening Exercises

STRAIGHT LEG PRESS

TARGETS:

» Muscles: Buttocks, hamstrings, back extensors.

» Bones: Hip and spine.

STARTING POSITION:

» Lie on your back and place your arms out from your side with your palms up and your knees bent.

» Straighten your right leg until it is resting on floor with toes and forefoot pulled towards your knee.

» Inhale using your diaphragm.

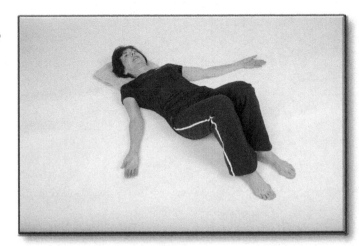

MOVEMENT:

Exhale and gently tighten your lower tummy as you:

» Squeeze your right buttock and press your right leg downward into floor.

» Keep the small of your back a hand-width from the floor.

» Hold for 2 to 3 seconds. Repeat 5 times.

» Be mindful to keep your neck in the lengthened position.

» Return your right leg to the start position. Then repeat with your left leg.

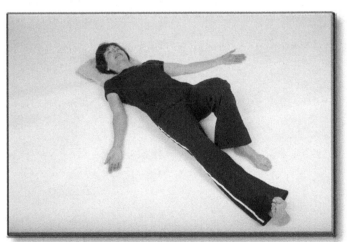

Postural Strengthening Exercises

7. Flexibility Exercises

Flexibility is an important component of bone health. The flexibility exercises presented in this chapter will not onto themselves help you build bone. They will, however, provide you with the range of motion you need to maintain a good posture and move with safe body mechanics.

Good flexibility will allow you to perform your strength and balance exercises and more importantly, your every day activities with more ease. This in turn will reduce the stress you place on your spine.

Once you begin strengthening a muscle you may find that your muscles tighten up. I encourage you to periodically go through the stretches presented in this chapter as a way of evaluating your own flexibility.

Tight quadriceps and hip flexors can lead to knee pain especially during lunges. Tight hamstring and calf muscles will limit your ability to bend safely from your hips. Tight neck, chest and latissimus dorsi muscles will pull you into a hunched back position.

If you are not flexible, your range of motion will be restricted and you could find that you will have to compromise your body position. As a result, I always include a flexibility assessment when I take on any new clients. If their flexibility is not where it should be, I encourage them to incorporate flexibility exercises into their program.

The flexibility exercises in this chapter are appropriate for all of the Exercise Levels. They can be used by you regardless of whether you were assigned a Beginner, Active, Athletic, or Elite Level Exercise Program.

I have made a point of selecting flexibility exercises that will allow you to build your flexibility without putting you at risk of a fracture.

As you go through the flexibility exercises in this chapter you will soon realize whether you need to do them or not. If you can perform the stretches with ease you need not spend too much time on this area. You should instead allocate your time to the later chapters dedicated to cardiovascular, strength, and balance for your level.

Finally, before you start the recommended flexibility exercises in this chapter, I have a number of very important flexibility tips I would like you to review:

» Stiffness around your ankle joint will increase your risk for falling – so make sure you keep your ankles flexible.

» A "bouncing" type of stretch will increase your risk of injury. Avoid flexibility exercises that incorporate bouncing.

» Breathing in a slow relaxed manner will help you get a more effective stretch.

» On a scale of 0 to 10 (with 10 being maximum discomfort and 0 being no stretch), you should stretch at a level of 5 to 7.

» Hold each stretch for 1 to 2 seconds, repeating the full movement ten times. If you are doing your stretches at the end of a workout, you may hold the last stretch for up to 3 minutes.

» If you want to increase your flexibility, you should do your stretching exercises every day.

» When you're satisfied with your level of flexibility, you can reduce your stretching to twice a week.

» Remember that loss of range of movement and muscle flexibility is different for each joint. Stretch where you feel tight or are not able to go through the full movement as demonstrated.

With all flexibility exercises (sometimes referred to as "stretches") I have indicated where you should feel the stretch. This is to help you relax into the stretch knowing you are doing the correct movement.

Good luck with building your flexibility.

QUADRICEPS STRETCH – STANDING

WHERE YOU SHOULD FEEL IT:

» Front of your thigh down to your kneecap.

STARTING POSITION:

» Stand tall in front of a chair.

» Place your hands on a steady surface for balance.

» Place one foot on the chair behind you.

» Inhale.

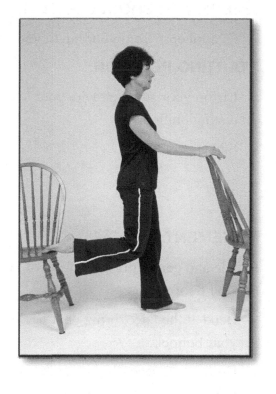

MOVEMENT:

Exhale and tighten your lower tummy as you:

» Draw your shoulders back over your hips.

» You can further increase the stretch by slowly bending the leg you are standing on.

» Hold for 1 to 2 seconds, straighten your leg and repeat 10 times before you go to the other side.

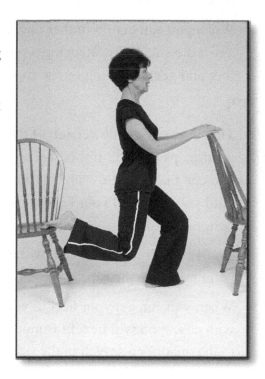

Flexibility Exercises

QUADRICEPS STRETCH – ON YOUR STOMACH

WHERE YOU SHOULD FEEL IT:

» Quadriceps (from your hip to your kneecap).

STARTING POSITION:

» Lie on your stomach with your legs straight, resting on floor.

» Inhale.

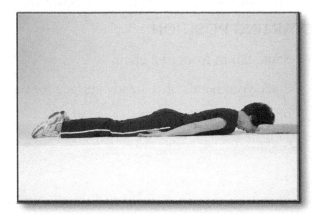

MOVEMENT:

Exhale and gently press the front of your pelvis into the floor as you:

» Bend at the knee, bring your heel towards your buttock.

» Hold 1 to 2 seconds and return. Repeat 10 times.

» When you can get no further on your own, assist the stretch by attaching a rope to your foot and gently pulling on the rope.

TIP:

» This is a very gentle version of the quadriceps stretch. If it is still too intense, you can place a pillow under your pelvis until you can bend your knee as shown in the bottom photo.

» Go back to doing the stretch without a pillow before you use the rope.

» When you can get your heel to your buttock with ease, you will benefit from progressing to the quadricep stretch in the side lying position (the next exercise).

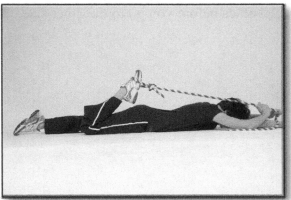

Flexibility Exercises

QUADRICEPS STRETCH – LYING ON YOUR SIDE

WHERE YOU SHOULD FEEL IT:

» Quadriceps (front thigh – from your hip to your kneecap).

STARTING POSITION:

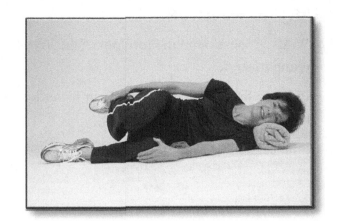

» Lie on your side with your knees pulled up towards your chest.

» Support your head with a pillow or rolled towel.

» Secure your bottom knee with your bottom hand.

» Grasp ankle of top leg with hand.

» Inhale.

MOVEMENT:

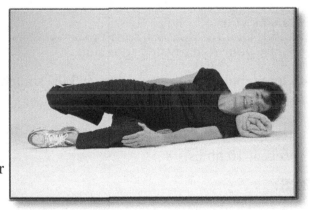

Exhale and gently tighten your lower tummy as you:

» Bring your leg in a backward direction.

» As you bring the top leg back think about squeezing your buttock allowing the front of your thigh (quadriceps) to stretch.

» Gently assist the movement by pulling on your ankle with your hand.

» Hold 1 to 2 seconds and return to start position. Repeat 10 times.

TIP:

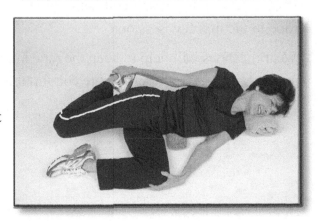

» Keep your knee (of the leg being stretched) at the height of your hip.

Flexibility Exercises

CALF STRETCH

WHERE YOU SHOULD FEEL IT:

» Gastrocnemius (calf).

STARTING POSITION:

» Wrap a rope around the forefoot of the leg you are going to stretch.

» Lie on a firm surface and rest your lower leg on a ball or pillow.

» Inhale.

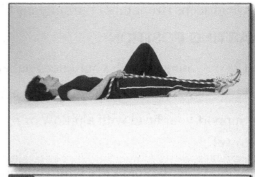

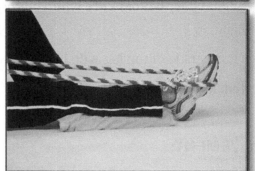

MOVEMENT:

Exhale as you:

» Draw your foot toward your shin.

» Gently pull the rope until you feel the stretch through your calf.

» Hold 1 to 2 seconds and return to start position. Repeat 10 times.

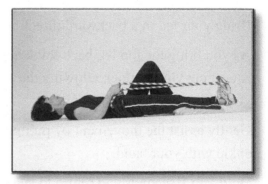

TIPS:

» If you are very tight, you will not need to use a rope in the first few sessions.

» Wearing shoes will help to keep the rope in place and may make the exercise more comfortable.

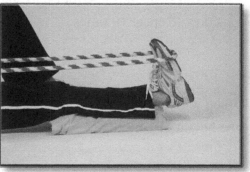

Flexibility Exercises

HAMSTRING STRETCH PART 1 – LOWER HAMSTRINGS

WHERE YOU SHOULD FEEL IT:

» Hamstrings (back of your thigh – to back of your knee).

STARTING POSITION:

» Wrap a rope around the arch of the foot you are going to stretch.

» Bring your knee toward your chest.

» Inhale.

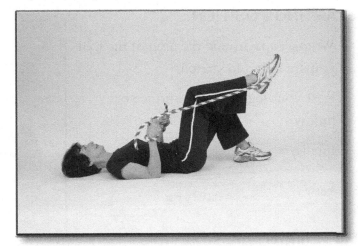

MOVEMENT:

Exhale as you:

» Straighten your knee.

» You will have to adjust the position of your thigh so that you feel a stretch in the back of your thigh when your knee is straightened.

» Assist the stretch by gently pulling on the rope.

» Hold 1 to 2 seconds and return to start position. Repeat 10 times.

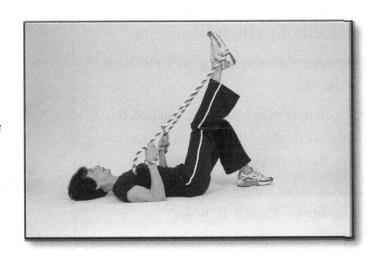

TIP:

» If you are unable to fully straighten your knee, then you should start with your knee lower before you straighten your knee.

Flexibility Exercises

HAMSTRING STRETCH PART 2 – UPPER HAMSTRINGS

WHERE YOU SHOULD FEEL IT:

» Hamstrings (back of your thigh – close to buttocks).

STARTING POSITION:

» Wrap a rope around the arch of the foot you are going to stretch.

» Rest your leg on a firm surface or pillow.

» Inhale.

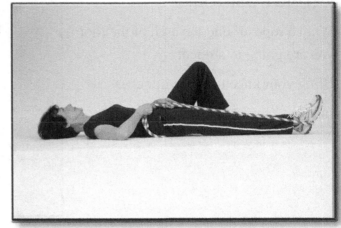

MOVEMENT:

Exhale and gently tighten your lower tummy as you:

» Lift your leg (your leg should be straight throughout movement).

» Assist the stretch by gently pulling on the rope.

» You may also place one hand on the upper thigh of the leg you are stretching to help keep your knee straight.

» Hold 1 to 2 seconds and return to start position. Repeat 10 times.

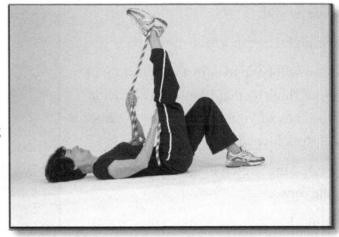

Flexibility Exercises

ILIOPSOAS STRETCH – KNEELING

WHERE YOU SHOULD FEEL IT:

» Iliopsoas (front of your hip).

» Upper thigh.

STARTING POSITION:

» On a soft surface, go into a half-kneeling position.

» Use a bench or chair for support.

» Maintain a tall posture with your hips and chest facing forward.

» Inhale.

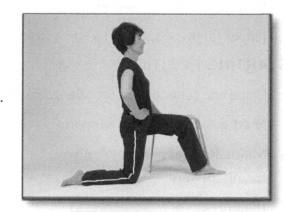

MOVEMENT:

Exhale and gently tighten your lower tummy as you:

» Draw you pelvis forward.

» Squeeze the buttock of the back leg.

» Keep your head and shoulders over your hips.

» Hold 1 to 2 seconds and return to starting position. Repeat 10 times.

» Repeat on opposite side.

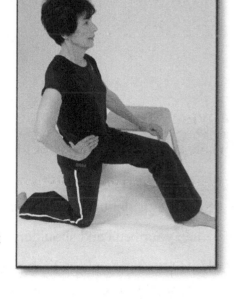

TIP:

» If you find the half-kneeling position uncomfortable, you can also stretch this muscle in standing.

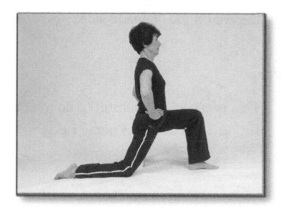

Flexibility Exercises

ILIOPSOAS STRETCH – STANDING

WHERE YOU SHOULD FEEL IT:

» Iliopsoas (front of your hip).

» Upper thigh.

STARTING POSITION:

» Place one foot on the seat of a stable chair.

» Hold the side chair for support.

» Maintain a tall posture with your hips and chest facing forward.

» Inhale.

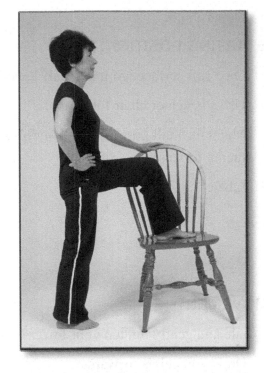

MOVEMENT:

Exhale and tighten your lower tummy as you:

» Draw you pelvis forward.

» Squeeze the buttock of the back leg.

» Keep your head and shoulders over your hips.

» Hold 1 to 2 seconds and return to starting position. Repeat 10 times.

» Repeat on the opposite side.

TIP:

» This is especially helpful to do after long periods of sitting, such as car or plane rides.

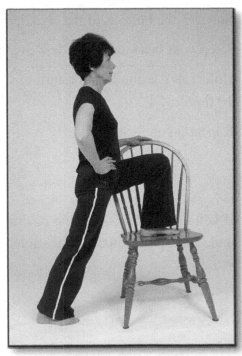

Flexibility Exercises

CHEST STRETCH – DOORWAY

WHERE YOU SHOULD FEEL IT:

» Chest and upper arms.

STARTING POSITION:

» Standing in a doorway place your forearms against the frame with your arms at 90 degrees.

» Step into the room maintaining good posture. You should not feel a stretch.

» Inhale.

MOVEMENT:

Exhale and tighten your lower tummy as you:

» Transfer your weight to the front foot.

» As you begin to feel a stretch lift your arms off the door frame so that you are making your back muscles do the work and not just hanging on your arms.

» Hold 1 to 2 seconds. Repeat 10 times.

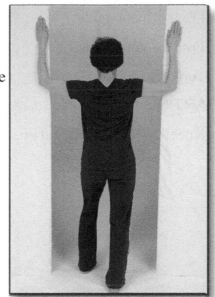

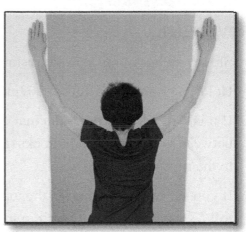

Repeat this exercise with your arms raised at 45 degrees from your last position as illustrated in the photo to the immediate right.

Flexibility Exercises

ANKLE STRETCH

WHERE YOU SHOULD FEEL IT:

» Front of your ankle.

» Front of your shins.

» Top of your feet.

STARTING POSITION:

» Kneel on your hands and knees.

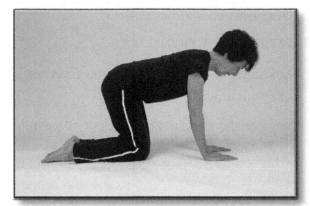

MOVEMENT:

» Slowly sit back until you are resting on your heels.

» Hold 1 to 2 seconds. Repeat 10 times.

» If it is difficult for you, roll a mat or pillow and place it between your heels and buttocks (as illustrated in the photo to the right).

» If you are feeling a strain in the top of your foot, roll a small towel and place it in front of your ankle between your ankle and the floor.

» As you get more flexible you can gradually reduce the size of the supports under your ankle and buttocks.

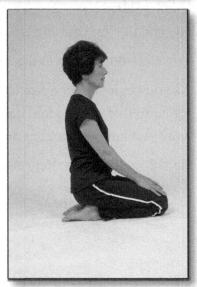

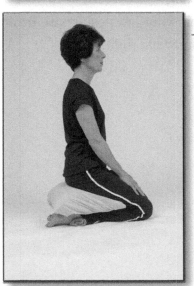

Flexibility Exercises

LAT STRETCH

WHERE YOU SHOULD FEEL IT:

» Latissimus dorsi (this runs from your pelvis to your upper arm).

» Quadratus lumborum (low back).

STARTING POSITION:

» Lie on a firm surface and slide your right leg to the left; secure it by resting your left ankle over top.

» Place your right hand beside your ear.

» Inhale.

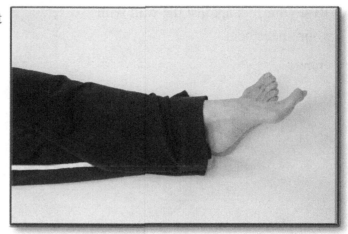

MOVEMENT:

Exhale as you:

» Slide your right hand across to the left bringing your body into a crescent shape.

» Hold for 1 to 2 seconds.

» Slide your right hand back by your ear and repeat the stretching movement 10 times.

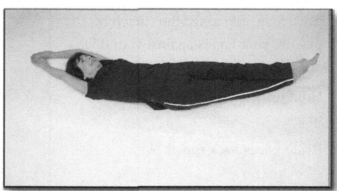

» Repeat the exercise on the opposite side.

» If this is uncomfortable on your shoulder, you can place a pillow above your head to rest your arms and/or bend at the elbows.

Flexibility Exercises

INNER THIGH STRETCH – BENT KNEES

WHERE YOU SHOULD FEEL IT:

» Inner thigh muscles.

STARTING POSITION:

» Lie on your back with your buttocks close to a wall.

» Rest your feet against the wall with your knees bent.

» Inhale.

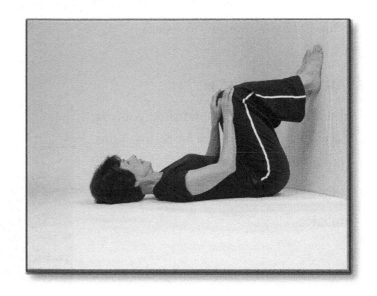

MOVEMENT:

Exhale and gently tighten your lower tummy as you:

» Spread your knees apart.

» You can gently assist the stretch by placing your hands against your thighs and press out further.

» Hold for 1 to 2 seconds. Repeat 10 times.

» Bring knees back together.

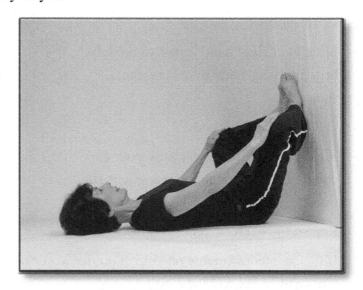

Flexibility Exercises

INNER THIGH STRETCH – STRAIGHT KNEES

WHERE YOU SHOULD FEEL IT:

» Inner thigh muscles.

START POSITION:

» Lie on your back with your buttocks within a foot of the wall.

» Wrap a rope around the leg you are going to stretch.

» Rest both legs up against the wall with your knees straight but not locked.

» Spread both legs a little from the midline.

» Inhale.

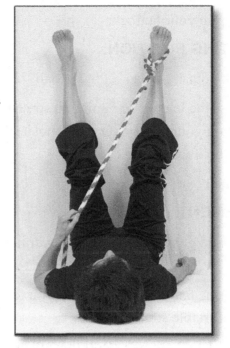

MOVEMENT:

Exhale and gently tighten your lower tummy as you:

» Slide the leg that is roped away from the other leg until you feel a comfortable stretch.

» Hold 1 to 2 seconds.

» Use the rope to assist you in bringing the stretched leg back to the starting position.

» Repeat 10 times and then perform the stretch on the opposite side.

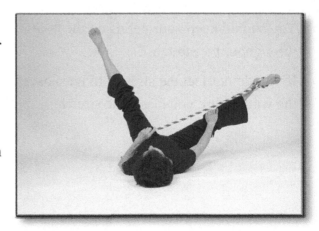

Flexibility Exercises

HIP ROTATOR STRETCH

WHERE YOU SHOULD FEEL IT:

» Outside of your hip.

» Deep in your buttock.

STARTING POSITION:

» Rest your legs over a Physio ball.

» Cross the leg you are going to stretch by resting your ankle over the opposite thigh – just below the knee.

» Inhale.

MOVEMENT:

Exhale and gently tighten your lower tummy as you:

» Roll the ball toward you until you feel a comfortable stretch.

» Hold 1 to 2 seconds. Roll the ball away. Repeat 10 times.

TIPS

» You should keep your pelvis on the floor throughout the stretch.

» If you do not feel the stretch, move closer to the wall before you begin the stretch.

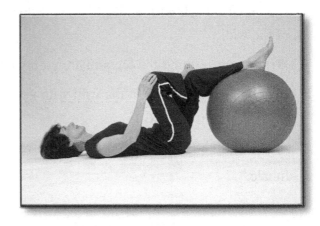

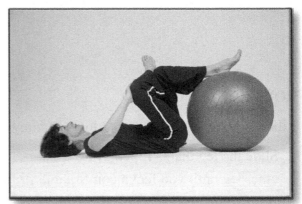

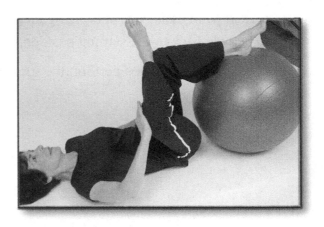

Flexibility Exercises

SPINAL STRETCH

WHERE YOU SHOULD FEEL IT:

» Abdominal muscles.

» Spine.

STARTING POSITION:

» Lie on your stomach, forehead resting on hands with elbows facing outward, palms down.

» Tuck your chin slightly.

» Inhale.

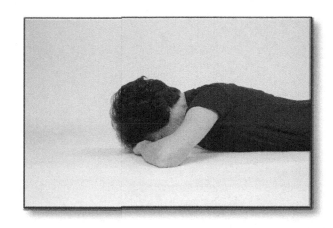

MOVEMENT:

Exhale and gently press the front of your pelvis into the floor as you:

» Tuck both elbows into your side, coming to rest directly under your shoulders.

» Relax into the stretch as you try to get your breastbone parallel to the wall in front of you.

» Hold 1 to 2 seconds and return to your start position.

» Repeat 10 times.

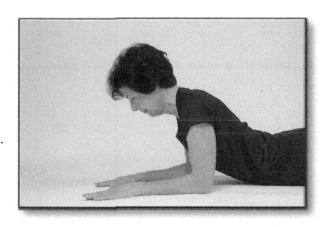

TIPS:

» Visualize your breast-bone parallel to the wall in front of you.

» Keep your gaze between your fingertips and the wall in front of you.

» If you find this stretch to be difficult or you feel discomfort in your low back, you should begin by using one to two pillows under your pelvis. As you regain your flexibility, you may reduce the size (and number) of the pillows until you can do this without any support from pillows.

Flexibility Exercises

8. Cardiovascular Exercises

Cardiovascular exercise is an important part of your bone health program. A bone friendly cardiovascular exercise program will not only allow you to maintain good aerobic health and keep your weight in check, it will also include activities that strengthen your bone structure. I want you to think about your cardiovascular training as a time to build your bones as well as your heart.

To strengthen your bones, you need to include cardiovascular activities that involve weight-bearing. Weight-bearing means that you are distributing the weight of your body through your skeleton. However, there are some activities that provide more weight-bearing benefit than others. This chapter will present the activities that maximize weight-bearing while taking into consideration your fracture risk level.

As we get older, we must find a balance between building stronger bones and being kind to our joints. We can do this by varying your workouts between high impact and lesser impact activities. The benefit of this approach is that it will help maintain your joint health as well as your bone health, and you will introduce variety into your exercise program so that you do not become bored over time and lose interest.

Remember that the cardiovascular component of your exercise program can take you outside the gym and into a set of activities that are social, fun, and stimulating. Yes, you can have fun and build aerobic and bone health at the same time!

To achieve maximum cardiovascular benefit, any physical activity that elevates your heart into its training range (your recommended training range is discussed on the next page) and sustains it for twenty continuous minutes, three times per week, is an appropriate minimum level of exercise.

Cardiovascular/weight-bearing recommendations have been categorized based on your fracture risk. Refer back to "Determining Your Fracture Risk Level" in Chapter 2 if you do not recall your fracture risk. I have provided you plenty of choices between activities and sports that provide the most weight-bearing to those that provide the least.

But before we get to the actual recommended cardiovascular exercises, I would like to discuss your recommended heart training range with you.

DETERMINE YOUR TRAINING RANGE

Use the Karvonen formula to determine your recommended heart rate exercise range (RHRER) for cardiovascular exercise.

First, determine your resting heart rate (RHR). The best time to take your resting heart rate is first thing in the morning before you do anything (even before getting out of bed, if possible). Count the number of heartbeats during a 15-second interval and multiply this number by 4. This result is the resting heart rate measured in number of beats per minute. For example, if you counted 18 heart beats during the 15-second interval, your resting heart rate (RHR) would be 72 beats per minute (i.e., 4 x 18 = 72).

Second, determine your maximum heart rate (MHR) by subtracting your age from 220. For example, a 65 year old would have a maximum heart rate (MHR) of 155 as shown here:

» 220 – age = 220 – 65 = 155 = MHR

Third, determine your heart rate reserve (HRR) by subtracting your resting heart rate (RHR) from your maximum heart rate (MHR). This will give you your Heart Rate Reserve (HRR). For example, our 65 year old above would have a heart rate reserve (HRR) of 83:

» HRR = MHR - RHR = 155 - 72 = 83

Finally, in order to find your recommended heart rate exercise range (RHRER) you must first multiply your heart rate reserve (HRR) by 60% and add back your resting heart rate (RHR). This will give you the low end of your recommended heart rate exercise range (RHRER). To determine your high end of your recommended heart rate exercise range (RHRER) multiply your heart rate reserve (HRR) by 85% and add back your resting heart rate (RHR).

» Low end RHRER: (60% of HRR) + RHR = (0.60 X 83) + 72 = 122 beats per minute

» High end RHRER: (85% of HRR) + RHR = (0.85 X 83) + 72 = 143 beats per minute

Therefore, the recommended heart rate exercise rate range (RHRER) for our 65 year old is between 122 and 143 beats per minute. You should repeat this every 8 weeks or so as you become more fit.

LOW FRACTURE RISK CARDIOVASCULAR EXERCISES

The low fracture risk category has no restrictions placed on it as far as the sport/activities you choose. Your first choice for a cardiovascular exercise that has maximum bone building benefit would be to choose from the following high impact weight-bearing activities:

» Soccer

» Hockey

» Volleyball

» Basketball

» Gymnastics

» Tennis

» Racquetball

» Martial arts

Your second choice for a cardiovascular exercise that has moderate bone building benefit would be to choose from the following moderate impact, weight-bearing, activities:

» Running/hiking

» Brisk walking

» Jumping rope

» Exerstriding/Nordic walking (brisk pace)

» Stair climbing

» Jogging on a treadmill/paths

» Stair-step machines

» Cross country skiing (brisk pace)

» Aerobics/step class

» Dancing (either line, square, tap – or all of them!)

» Tai Chi

» Circuit training

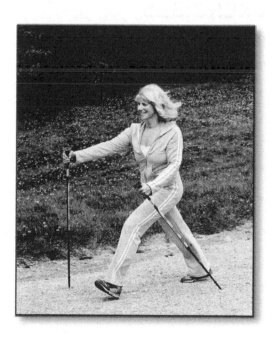

Cardiovascular Exercises

Your third choice for a cardiovascular exercise that has minimum bone building benefit would be to choose from the following low impact weight-bearing activities:

» Walking at a leisurely pace

» Swimming

» Deep-water walking

» Water aerobics

» Low impact aerobics

» Exerstriding/Nordic walking (leisurely pace)

» Cross-country ski machines (moderate pace)

» Cross-country skiing (moderate pace)

» Therapeutic exercise classes

» Elliptical machine

» Cycling

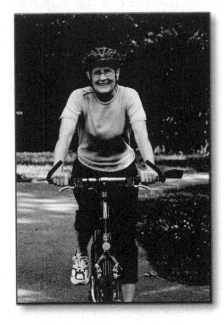

MODERATE FRACTURE RISK CARDIOVASCULAR EXERCISES

If you are in the moderate fracture risk category it is important that you choose activities that maximize loading but do not require a lot of rotation and forward flexion. Your first choice for a cardiovascular exercise that has maximum bone building benefit would be to choose from the following moderate impact weight-bearing activities:

» Running/hiking

» Brisk walking

» Jumping rope

» Exerstriding/Nordic walking (brisk pace)

» Stair climbing

» Jogging on a treadmill/paths

» Stair-step machines

» Cross country skiing (brisk pace)

» Aerobics/step class

» Dancing (line, tap, square)

Cardiovascular Exercises

» Circuit training

Your second choice for a cardiovascular exercise that has moderate bone building benefit would be to choose from the following moderate/low impact weight-bearing activities:

» Water aerobics/aqua fit

» Low impact aerobics

» Tai Chi

» Walking moderate pace

» Exerstriding/Nordic walking (moderate pace)

» Therapeutic exercise classes.

» Elliptical machine

» Dancing (ballroom)

Your third choice for a cardiovascular exercise that has minimum bone building benefit would be to choose from the following low impact weight-bearing activities:

» Indoor cycling

» Therapeutic aqua fit

» Walking leisurely pace

» Exerstriding/Nordic walking (leisurely pace)

» Cross-country ski machines (moderate pace)

HIGH FRACTURE RISK CARDIOVASCULAR EXERCISES

If you are in the high fracture risk it is important that you choose activities that do not place you at risk for a fall or which are too aggressive. Your first choice for a cardiovascular exercise that has maximum bone building benefit would be to choose from the following moderate impact weight-bearing activities:

» Brisk walking

» Exerstriding/Nordic walking (brisk pace)

» Stair climbing/stair step machine

» Dancing (line, square, tap)

» Low impact aerobics

» Tai Chi

» Circuit training

Your second choice for a cardiovascular exercise that has moderate bone building benefit would be to choose from the following moderate/low impact weight-bearing activities:

» Walking at moderate pace

» Swimming

» Deep-water walking/running

» Aqua fit/ Water aerobics

» Exerstriding/Nordic walking (moderate pace)

» Therapeutic exercise classes

» Elliptical machine (moderate to brisk pace)

» Cross country ski machine (moderate to brisk pace)

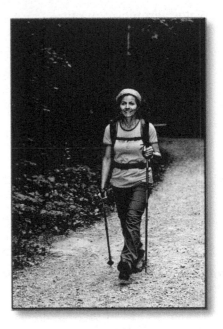

Your third choice for a cardiovascular exercise that has minimum bone building benefit would be to choose from the following low impact weight-bearing activities:

» Indoor cycling

» Therapeutic aqua fit

» Walking at leisurely pace

» Exerstriding/Nordic walking (leisurely pace)

Cardiovascular Exercises

RECOVERING FROM A FRAGILITY FRACTURE

If you are recovering from a fragility fracture you should consult with your Physician or your Physical Therapist regarding your exercise program. I encourage my clients who are recovering from a fragility fracture to be active. The following exercises are safe for people who are recovering from a fragility fracture.

» Swimming (backstroke encouraged)

» Therapeutic exercise class

» Deep water walking or running

» Indoor cycling with handle bars positioned by the seat

» Therapeutic aqua fit

» Tai Chi

THERAPEUTIC / SENIOR EXERCISE CLASSES

If possible, avoid doing exercises in a seated position as it places more compression on your spine than exercising in a standing position. Avoid all exercises that involve bending forward (such as touching your toes). Ensure that the instructor is educated about Osteoporosis. Only do the exercises you know are safe for you.

CARDIOVASCULAR EXERCISE CONSIDERATIONS

The last thing that you want to see happen is that you are diligent and follow an exercise program only to find out that you caused a fracture because of poor form. Remember that there are exercise activities that you should modify or avoid altogether. You will find my recommended exercise guidelines in Chapter 4 – Exercise Tips and Chapter 5 – Exercises to Avoid.

SWIMMING

Swimming is an excellent cardiovascular activity. However, it is not as effective at bone building as the weight-bearing exercises listed earlier in this chapter. If swimming is an activity that you like to do, here are my suggestions regarding what you should do when you are in the water:

» Do not only do front crawl. It tends to encourage a rounded back.

» Do plenty of backstroke, breaststroke, sidestroke, and legwork.

9. Beginner Level Strength Exercises

By now you should have read and completed the foundation chapters in this guide. You should be comfortable with your bone and body basics (Chapter 3), know the key exercise safety tips (Chapter 4), understand which exercises and poses you should avoid and why (Chapter 5), have optimized your posture (Chapter 6), have checked your flexibility (Chapter 7), and have selected the cardiovascular exercises are right for you (Chapter 8).

You should have determined your appropriate Exercise level. Your activity level will be either Beginner, Active, Athletic, or Elite, and your fracture risk will be either Low, Moderate, or High (see Chapter 2).

Since you are reading the Beginner Level Exercise chapter, I am assuming that you have selected the Beginner Level. The Beginner Level Exercise program is designed for people who are either at a low, moderate, or high fracture risk, and who have not done any exercises in months, years, or ever – other than light housekeeping or gardening.

Be sure to download your Exercise Plan at **www.melioguide.com/exercise-plans** and have it in hand.

There are two major exercise sections in this chapter. The Beginner Level Exercises are categorized into Warm Up and Strength. As you progress through the chapter, the type of exercise (Warm Up, Strength) will be indicated at the bottom of each page.

The Cardiovascular, Flexibility, and Postural Exercises have been covered in earlier chapters. Please refer to these chapters for more detail.

The frequency and progression of the **Warm Up** and **Strength** exercises should be followed as described in your Exercise Plan. For the Strength exercises you will require dumbbells, an exercise mat or comfortable carpet to lie on, and an elastic band. The equipment you will need can be found at most major outlet stores. If you feel any discomfort with any of the exercises, you should consult with a Physical Therapist before proceeding further.

Before you start, let me clarify what I mean in the Exercise Plan when I say "sets" and "reps." **Reps** is an abbreviation for repetitions. This is the number of repetitions you do before your muscles are too tired to do any more. Thus, if I ask you to do a set of ten repetitions, I want you to pick a weight that makes the exercise hard enough that by the tenth repetition the muscle you are targeting is very fatigued and you would have a hard time completing another repetition with good form. If the recommended second set indicates that you perform fewer repetitions than the first set, then you should choose a heavier weight or slow down your cadence.

Sets represent the number of times you redo the exercise. If I ask you to do two sets you should not do them back-to-back. The muscle being targeted needs time to recover – a full minute at the very least!

This doesn't mean you have to sit around and wait. Your recovery time can be used working another muscle group or working on your Balance exercises. I designed the exercise series so that you could do them one after another. This approach allows for an active recovery period. This saves you time and builds a cardiovascular component into your program.

Under the Strength Exercises I have listed the main muscles involved in executing the exercise as well as which part of your skeleton gets the most stimulation from the exercise. The three most frequent bone fracture areas (spine, hip, and wrist) are identified. The muscle groups and affected bones are listed under "Targets."

For example, while doing a squat, your muscles at the front of your thighs and your buttocks are the most active and your hip bones are loaded. Your spine gets loaded as you hold your chest forward, hold a weight, or wear a weighted vest while doing your squat.

Use of Affirmations During the Warm Up Exercises

You should use personal affirmations as you go through your Warm Ups to start your session off on the right foot and get yourself into the right frame of mind. An affirmation is a positive personal thought. As you inhale, say to yourself "I am." As you exhale, choose an affirmation to take with you into your workout: "energized"… "balanced" ... "strong" .... "focussed". Now onto your first Warm Up Exercise.

WARM UP 1 – ENERGY TREE

STARTING POSITION:

» Stand tall.

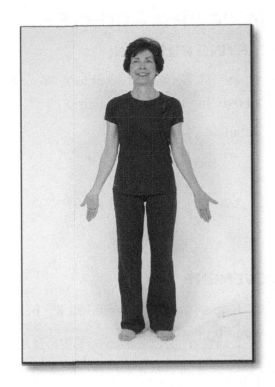

MOVEMENT:

» Inhale as you as you raise arms overhead, lifting your rib cage up – gathering energy as you reach to the sky.

» Exhale as you bring your arms by your side, keeping your rib cage lifted.

» Repeat.

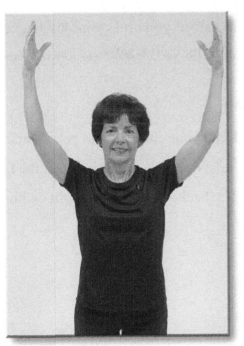

Beginner Warm Up Exercises

WARM UP 2 – CURTSEY

STARTING POSITION:

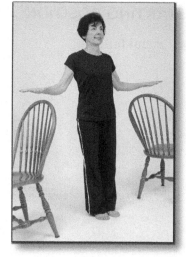

» Stand tall between two chairs. Your hands should be resting above, but not on, the chairs.

» Inhale.

MOVEMENT:

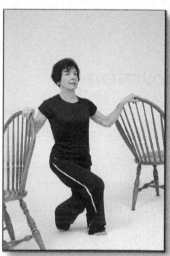

» Exhale as you cross your left leg behind your right leg, gently bending both knees.

» Return to start position by pushing your front foot into the floor. Inhale.

» Exhale as you cross your left leg behind your right, gently bending both knees.

TIPS:

» Keep your chest up and pelvis facing forward.

» Most of the weight will be on the front leg.

» The heel of the back leg will be raised.

Beginner Warm Up Exercises

WARM UP 3 – MARCHING

STARTING POSITION:

» Stand tall.

MOVEMENT:

» March on the spot as you breathe in and out.

» Simultaneosly swing your opposite arm towards the ceiling as you march.

» Raise your knees as high as you comfortably can. If you feel unstable you should do this between two chairs.

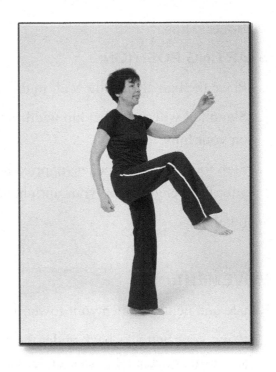

TIPS:

» If you are unsteady on your feet, stand between two chairs with your hands resting above them but not on them.

» Swinging your arms with a bent elbow will allow you to march at a quicker pace. This has good carryover for brisk walking.

Beginner Warm Up Exercises

WALL AND BALL SQUATS

TARGETS:

» Muscles: Quadriceps, buttocks.

» Bones: Hips.

STARTING POSITION:

» Place the ball against the wall in the small of your back.

» Stand tall with your feet hip width apart, hands resting on your hips.

» Step forward 4 to 6 inches (approximately a half of your foot length) from your upright position.

» Inhale.

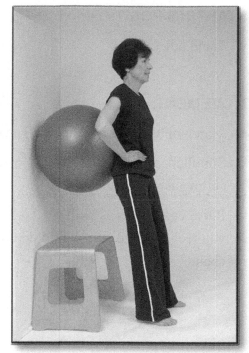

MOVEMENT:

Exhale and gently tighten your lower tummy as you:

» Bring your buttocks back under the ball as though you are sitting on a stool placed under the ball.

» Return to standing position and repeat movement until set is completed.

TIPS:

» Keep the middle of your knee cap pointing in the same direction as your second toe.

» Only go as far as you can comfortably go. With time, you will be able to get into a seated position with your thighs parallel to the floor.

» Squeeze your buttocks and push the floor away from you as you return to your standing position.

» As you squat, the ball will move to your mid and upper back region and your weight should be evenly distributed between your heel and forefoot. Keep your eyes facing forward.

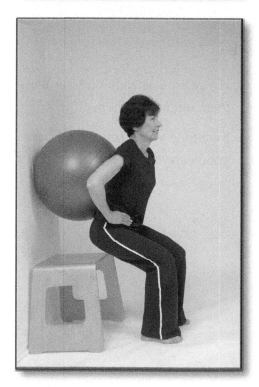

Beginner Strength Exercises

REVERSE FLY

TARGETS:

» Muscles: Middle and upper back.

» Bones: Spine.

STARTING POSITION:

» Stand with your buttocks, upper back and the back of your head against the wall. Keep your chin tucked in and eyes facing forward.

» Your heels should be four to six inches from the wall, your knees slightly bent.

» Hold the TheraBand band allowing roughly 12 to 18 inches of band between hands.

» Inhale as you raise your arms to shoulder height with your thumbs pointing to the ceiling.

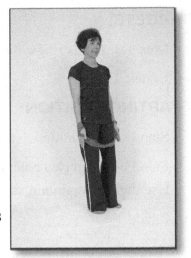

MOVEMENT:

Exhale and gently tighten your lower tummy as you:

» Squeeze your shoulder blades together as you bring your arms back.

» Return in a controlled manner to starting position and repeat until set is completed.

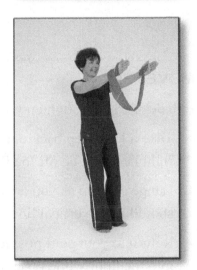

TIPS:

» To ease into this exercise, you can bring one arm back at a time.

» You should have no more than a hand-sized space in the small of your back throughout this exercise.

» Adjust the length of the band between your hands to get the resistance you need.

» Refer to "Wrapping the TheraBand" in Chapter 4. This is especially important if you have arthritic hands.

» If your head does not rest easily against the wall hold a rolled face cloth between your head and the wall.

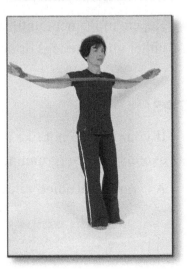

Beginner Strength Exercises

REVERSE LUNGE BETWEEN CHAIRS

TARGETS:

» Muscles: Hamstrings, buttocks, and quadriceps.

» Bones: Hips.

STARTING POSITION:

» Stand with an athletic stance.

» Stand between two chairs or a chair and a counter top. Use them to maintain stability.

» Inhale.

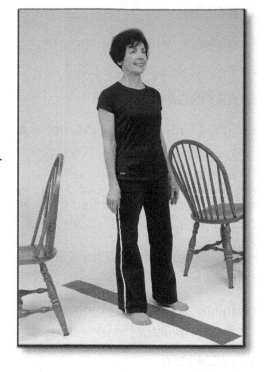

MOVEMENT:

Exhale and gently tighten your lower tummy as you:

» Take a long step back onto your right forefoot (your right heel will be off the floor).

» Lunge as deep as you are comfortable. Your right knee should be in vertical line with your hips and shoulders.

» Return to your start position by pressing your left leg into the floor while pushing off with your right foot.

» Repeat movement until your set is complete. You can either alternate legs or do all right and then all left.

TIPS:

» If your toes do not like the pressure, you may try this exercise wearing running shoes.

» As you get steadier, release the chair.

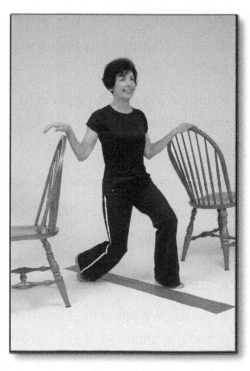

Beginner Strength Exercises

HORSE STANCE VERTICAL

TARGETS:

» Muscles: Deep back muscles.

» Bones: Spine and wrist.

STARTING POSITION:

» Assume a four-point kneeling position.

» Keep your knees directly under your hips and your hands directly under your shoulders.

» Keep your elbows unlocked and pointing towards your thighs.

» You should have a hand-width space in your low back. A yardstick along your spine helps to keep you in perfect alignment. Contact points should be your pelvis, mid-back, and back of your head.

» With your spine kept in a neutral alignment position, take a deep relaxed breath.

MOVEMENT:

Exhale and gently tighten your lower tummy as you:

» Begin transferring your weight off the limb to be lifted.

» Raise one hand slightly (enough to slide a sheet of paper between your hand and the floor).

» Hold this position for up to five seconds.

» Repeat this pattern with your opposite hand, your left leg and your right leg (one at a time!)

» Each individual lift corresponds to a single repetition on your Exercise Plan.

TIPS:

» Throughout the exercise, keep your spine motionless.

» If you are unable to tolerate resting on your wrist, you can do the exercise with your forearms on a small bench, or with a small towel rolled under your palms (but not your fingers).

Beginner Strength Exercises

BRIDGING

TARGETS:

» Muscles: Buttocks, hamstrings, and back.

» Bones: Hips and spine.

STARTING POSITION:

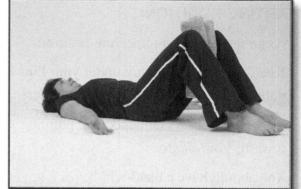

» Lie on your back, knees bent, knees and feet hip-width apart, arms out from your side with palms up.

» Squeeze a rolled towel or pillow between your knees.

» Inhale.

MOVEMENT:

Exhale as you:

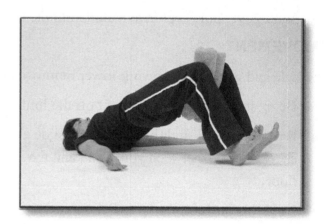

» Squeeze your buttocks and push down through your heels.

» Transfer your weight onto your shoulder blades as you lift your hips towards the ceiling.

» Raise your toes as you raise your hips, lowering your toes as you lower your hips.

» As you come down lengthen your spine as though your tail-bone is reaching towards your heels.

» Return in a controlled manner to starting position and repeat movement until set is completed.

TIP:

» You should feel this in your buttocks, back of your thighs, and muscles along your spine.

» Transfer your body weight to your heels and shoulder blades and not to the back of your neck.

» Go high enough that you are bringing your hips into the line drawn between your hips and shoulders.

Beginner Strength Exercises

BOW AND ARROW

TARGETS:

» Muscles: Upper and middle back.

» Bones: Spine.

STARTING POSITION:

» Stand with your buttocks, upper back, and the back of your head against the wall. Keep your chin tucked in and eyes facing forward.

» Your heels should be 4 to 6 inches from the wall, knees slightly bent.

» Hold the TheraBand band such that only 6 to 8 inches of band remains between your hands.

» Inhale as you raise your arms to shoulder height with your knuckles pointing to the ceiling.

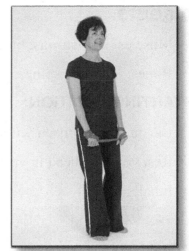

MOVEMENT:

Exhale and gently tighten your lower tummy as you:

» Pull your right elbow into the wall as you keep your left arm out as though holding a bow.

» Focus on your shoulder blade drawing towards your spine as you pull your elbow back.

» Return in a controlled manner to the starting position and repeat until set is completed.

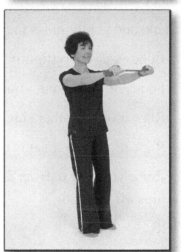

TIPS:

» You should have no more than a hand size space in the small of your back throughout this exercise.

» You may need to double up your TheraBand band for more resistance.

» You may return your arms down to your thighs in between each repetition.

» If your head does not rest easily against the wall hold a rolled face cloth between your head and the wall.

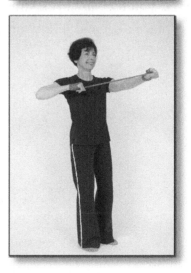

Beginner Strength Exercises

ALTERNATING LEG LIFTS – PRONE

TARGETS:

» Muscles: Hamstrings, buttocks, and lower back.

» Bones: Hips and spine.

STARTING POSITION:

» Lie on your stomach with a pillow under your pelvis.

» Rest your forehead in your palms.

» Inhale.

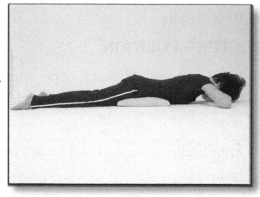

MOVEMENT:

Exhale and gently press the front of your pelvis into the pillow as you:

» Bend your knee slightly and lift your leg off the floor.

» Focus on squeezing your butt as you lift.

» Repeat on the other side.

» Repeat until your set is completed.

» Raise your leg only as far as you can without lifting hips off the floor.

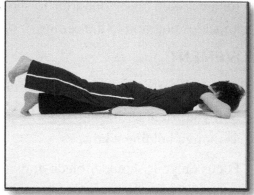

TIPS:

» If you feel any back strain with this exercise, you can place a second pillow under your pelvis.

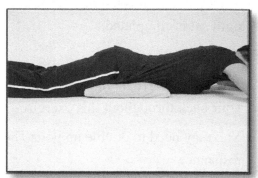

Beginner Strength Exercises

SIDE LYING LEG LIFTS

TARGETS:

» Muscles: Abductors (the muscles in your upper hip/buttocks).

» Bones: Hips.

STARTING POSITION:

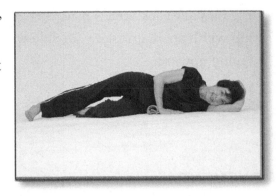

» Lie on your side against a wall with head, mid-back, pelvis, and heel of top leg in contact with wall.

» Bottom leg should be comfortably bent, foot against the wall.

» Your upper hip and knee should be straight but not locked.

» Rest your head on your bottom arm or a pillow.

» Inhale.

MOVEMENT:

Exhale and gently tighten your lower tummy as you:

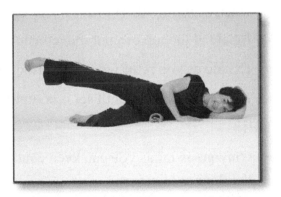

» Keep your heel in contact with the wall and slowly lift your top leg.

» Turn your kneecap and foot slightly to the ceiling as you lift and lower your leg (not shown).

» Repeat the movement until your set is completed.

» Switch leg and repeat movement.

TIPS:

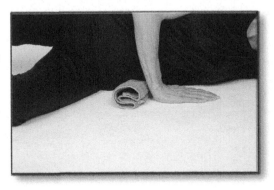

» If your hips are wider than your waist, you should place a small pillow or rolled towel in the space between your pelvis and rib cage as illustrated in the photo to the immediate right.

» Your top heel should remain in contact with the wall throughout the exercise.

Beginner Strength Exercises

ANGELS IN THE SNOW

TARGETS:

» Muscles: Back and shoulders.

» Bones: Spine.

STARTING POSITION:

» Lie on your back, knees bent, feet on floor hip width apart, arms at your side with palms facing upward.

» Inhale.

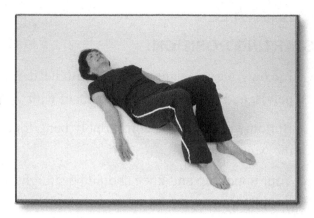

MOVEMENT:

Exhale and gently tighten your lower tummy as you:

» Press your upper arms into the floor and move both arms at the same time as though making angel wings in the snow.

» Inhale at the top of your movement.

» Exhale as you return to your starting position.

» Repeat movement until set is completed.

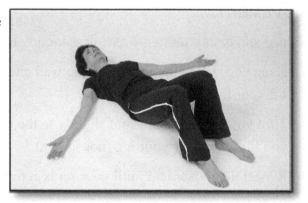

TIP:

» Only go as far as you can keep contact with the floor at all times.

» Be sure to press your upper arms (above your elbow) into the floor to ensure you are using your back muscles to do the movement.

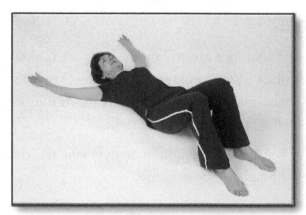

Beginner Strength Exercises

WALL PUSH UP

TARGETS:

» Muscles: Chest, triceps, and abdominals.

» Bones: Wrists and spine.

STARTING POSITION:

» Place your hands one and one-half shoulder width apart on the wall with your hands turned slightly towards each other.

» Stand far enough back to create a lean into the wall as if you were the Leaning Tower of Pisa.

» Inhale.

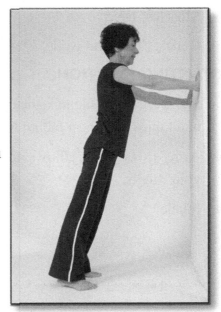

MOVEMENT:

Exhale and gently tighten your lower tummy as you:

» Lower your body towards the wall, bending your elbows away from you.

» Push away, straightening but not locking the elbows.

» Repeat movement.

TIPS:

» Keep your head, shoulders, hips and ankles in line throughout the exercise.

» Let yourself rock forward onto the balls of your feet, lifting your heels.

» If a wall pushup feels too easy, you can progress to a pushup from a counter top or the stairs. The lower the surface, the more challenging the exercise will become.

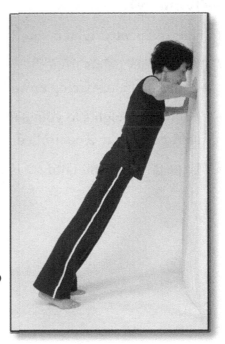

Beginner Strength Exercises

STANDING BICEPS CURL

TARGETS:

» Muscles: Biceps.

» Bones: Spine and wrists.

STARTING POSITION:

» Stand with an athletic stance with a weight in each hand, hips and chest facing forward.

» Arms at your side, elbows unlocked, palms facing your thighs.

» Inhale.

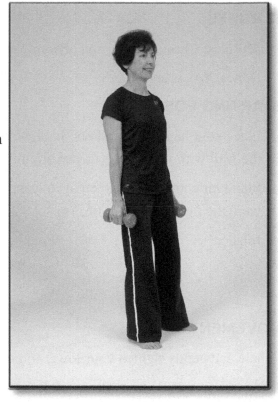

MOVEMENT:

Exhale and gently tighten your lower tummy as you:

» Move your palms from their start position, facing thighs, to palms facing upward.

» Bring the weights to your shoulders and return to start position in a controlled manner.

» Repeat movement until set is completed.

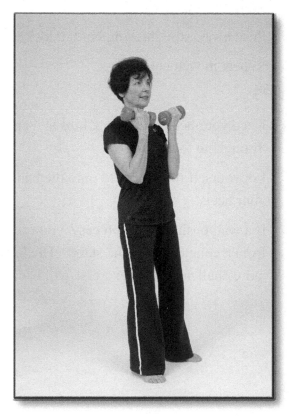

Beginner Strength Exercises

TRICEPS EXTENSION FROM FLOOR

TARGETS:

» Muscles: Triceps.

» Bones: Wrists.

STARTING POSITION:

» Lie on back, knees bent and feet on floor, knees and feet shoulder-width apart.

» Hold one weight in both hands with your arms straight and hands in line with forehead.

» Inhale.

MOVEMENT:

Exhale and gently tighten your lower tummy as you:

» Bend your elbows, lowering the weight until it almost reaches the floor behind you.

» Return to start position in controlled manner.

» Repeat the movement until set is completed.

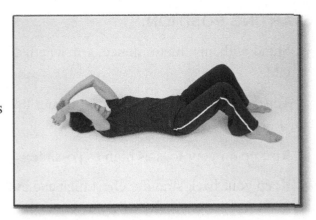

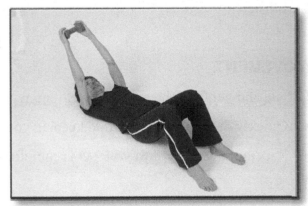

TIPS:

» Keep your shoulders and upper arms steady through the bending and straightening of your elbow.

» Do not lock your elbows.

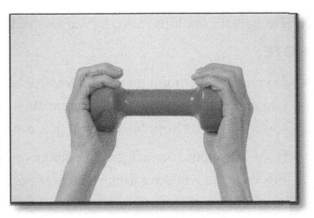

Beginner Strength Exercises

HEEL DROPS

TARGETS:

» Muscles: Calves.

» Bones: Hips.

STARTING POSITION:

» Stand with an athletic stance, arm length distance from the table.

» Touch the counter top lightly with your fingertips to balance yourself.

» Rise up on your toes as high as possible.

» Keep your back straight, chest high and eyes looking forward.

» Inhale.

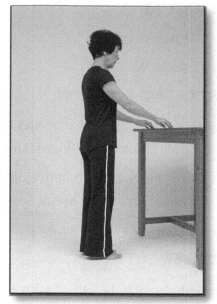

MOVEMENT:

Exhale and gently tighten your lower tummy as you:

» Quickly drop your heels while keeping your body tall.

» Repeat movement until your set is completed.

TIPS:

» Do not bend at the knees. Keep your legs straight but do not lock your knees.

» Do not let your hips move forward or backward.

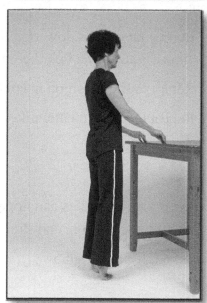

NOTE:

» If you have any joint pain in your lower body or have had a previous compression fracture, then you should lower gently on your heels rather than drop quickly.

» If you have pain or stiffness in your toes, you may do this exercise while wearing running shoes.

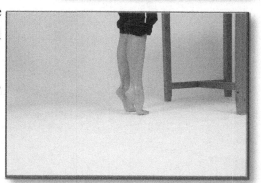

Beginner Strength Exercises

ABDOMINAL ACTIVATION

TARGETS:

» Muscles: Transverse abdominus.

» Bones: Spine.

STARTING POSITION:

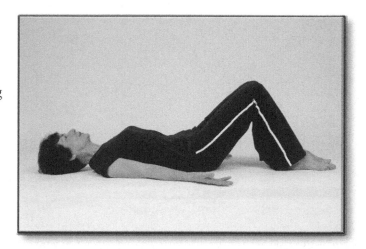

» Lie on floor with knees bent, feet and knees hip-width apart and arms resting out from your sides, palms up.

» Place a small rolled towel in the small of your back (roll should be the width and depth of your hand).

» Inhale with your diaphragm and relax your pelvic floor.

MOVEMENT:

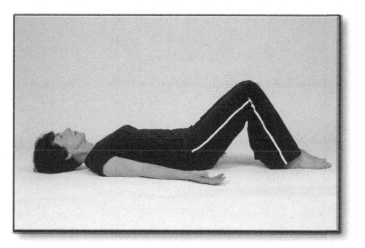

» As you exhale, slowly, gently tighten your pelvic floor muscles and your lower tummy.

» If you cannot feel your deep abdominal muscles tighten, I find that many of my clients are successful when I ask them to pull their pelvic bones together. The bones do not actually move, but the deep muscles will tighten.

» Hold for 5 seconds and relax.

» Repeat up to 10 times.

TIP:

» Please refer to "Pull in Your Tummy" for proper abdominal activation tips in Chapter 4 – Exercise Safety Tips.

Beginner Strength Exercises

10. Beginner Level Balance Exercises

Balance is a critical component of your exercise program. Balance becomes increasingly important as our bones age and become more fragile. We use our balance to keep us from falls that could lead to a fracture.

Increased balance allows you to be more independent and confident and can greatly affect the quality of your life. The more balanced you are when you perform day-to-day activities, the more likely you are to be active in life.

The balance exercises in this chapter have been developed for people who are either Low, Moderate, or High fracture risk.

These balance exercises will make you more stable and will have a direct impact on reducing your fracture risk. With practice, your balance will improve. Follow these instructions when you are performing your balance training:

» Choose among the exercises listed that challenge you.

» Make sure that you can hold your position for at least 10 seconds.

» Mix up the exercises from week to week for variety.

» Do a total of 3 to 5 minutes of balance training each session.

» Keep safety in mind by practicing your balance exercises in a safe location, such as a corner of a room with a sturdy chair in front of you for support.

» Maintain an athletic stance as discussed in Chapter 4.

BODY SWAY

There are two steps to this balance exercise. During the first step you will establish your stance and determine whether your are steady enough in this position to proceed to the second step. During the second step you will sway your body.

Let's start with establishing your stance:

» Stand between two chairs and place your feet together.

» Hold the two chairs.

» Let go of one of the chairs and then release your grip of the other chair. Hold this position for 20 seconds.

How did you feel during the 20 seconds you were standing without the support of the two chairs? If you did not feel completely steady and comfortable, then you should perform the body sway movements, described below, with your feet shoulder width apart.

The following are several body sway movements you should perform:

» Sway your body side to side. Keep your body straight and do not pick up your feet or bend your knees. Move as though you were a solid structure from your ankles to the top of your head.

» Sway your body forward and backward (onto the balls of your feet then onto your heels).

»

STEPPING

Stand between the two chairs and maintain your grip on both chairs. Take a full step forward. Let go of one chair and, when you are ready, let go of the other chair. Hold that position for up to 30 seconds.

Repeat with the other leg forward.

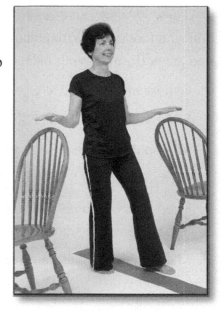

Beginner Balance Exercises

STEPPING ON THE LINE

Imagine you are a tight rope walker and that you are about to step onto the suspended line. Start this exercise by standing between the two chairs and maintaining a firm supportive grip on both chairs.

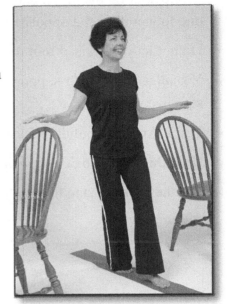

» Step forward with one of your feet onto the imaginary tight rope.

» Keep your feet several inches apart with one foot directly in front of the other (not shown in photos).

» Let go of one chair and then the other.

» Hold for up to 30 seconds.

» Repeat with the other leg forward.

» Now bring your feet closer together so that your heel of your forward foot is touching the toes on the back foot as illustrated in the photos.

Repeat with the other leg forward.

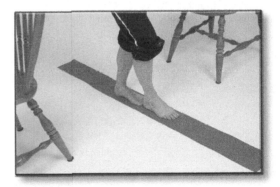

Beginner Balance Exercises

SINGLE LEG STANCE

Start this exercise by standing between the two chairs and maintaining a firm supportive grip on both chairs.

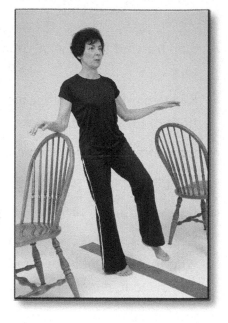

»   While holding the top of each chair, transfer your weight to one foot and lift the opposite foot.

»   Do not let your raised foot rest on your supporting leg.

»   Visualize filling your supporting leg with sand to help you stabilize yourself.

»   When you feel confident release one chair, then the other.

»   Hold this for up to 30 seconds with your eyes open.

Repeat the exercise standing on the opposite foot.

Beginner Balance Exercises

SINGLE LEG STANCE WITH MOVEMENT

While standing on one foot move the opposite leg in a slow, controlled manner. Move your elevated leg:

» Forward, returning your leg to the starting position after each movement.

» Sideways.

» Behind you.

Build up your endurance and balance to the point where you can comfortably repeat the sequence 6 times on each leg.

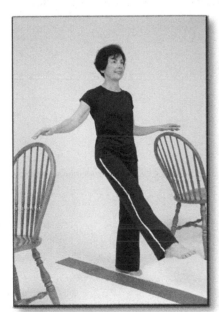 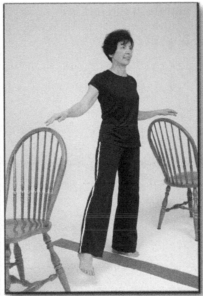 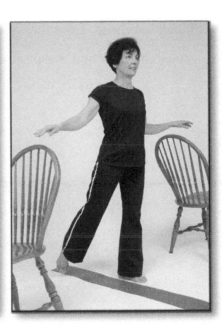

Beginner Balance Exercises

VARIATIONS

You can modify any of the beginner balance exercises and create new challenges for yourself. The following are several suggested modifications for you to incorporate into your balance exercises:

» Perform the exercises on a softer surface such as a thick carpet, an exercise mat, a half foam roller, out on the grass or in the sand!

» Keep your arms crossed in front of you.

» Turn your head from side to side.

» Look up and down.

» You can also train with a partner and toss a ball back and forth. You can toss the ball under hand, overhead, from the right, and from the left.

» You can cover one eye or close both eyes.

Beginner Balance Exercises

PHYSIO BALL BALANCE EXERCISE

The following exercise should only be done using the correct size ball that is marked "Burst Resistant". Please refer to the section Equipment Recommendations – Burst-Resistant Physio Ball in Chapter 1 for the correct type and size of Physio Ball.

You should also review "Safely Using a Physio Ball" in Chapter 4 – Exercise Safety Tips if you are unfamiliar with using a Physio Ball or if it has been a long time since you last were on one.

STARTING POSITION:

» Sit comfortably on the Physio Ball.

» Feet should be shoulder width apart.

» Have your knees bent to a right angle and your knees directly over your feet.

MOVEMENT:

» Shift your hips right and left as illustrated in the photos.

» Shift only as far as you are comfortable.

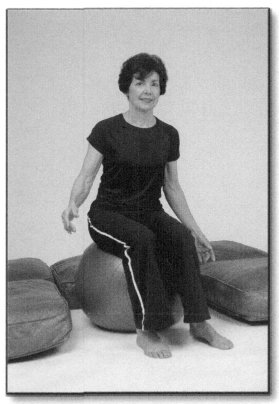

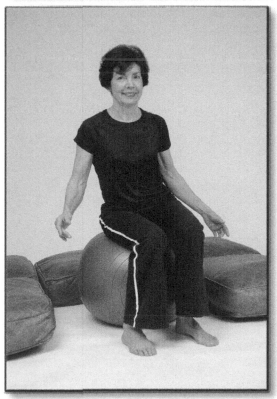

Beginner Balance Exercises

11. Active Level Strength Exercises

By now you should have read and completed the foundation chapters in this guide. You should be comfortable with your bone and body basics (Chapter 3), know the key exercise safety tips (Chapter 4), understand which exercises and poses you should avoid and why (Chapter 5), have optimized your posture (Chapter 6), have checked your flexibility (Chapter 7), and have selected the cardiovascular exercises are right for you (Chapter 8).

You should have determined your appropriate exercise level. Your activity level will be either Beginner, Active, Athletic, or Elite, and your fracture risk will be either Low, Moderate, or High (see Chapter 2).

Since you are reading the Active Level Exercise chapter, I am assuming that you have selected the Active Level. The Active Level Exercise program is designed for people who are either at a low, moderate, or high fracture risk, and who have been involved in a fairly regular exercise program (1 to 2 sessions per week) in the past six months. You do (or could do) all your own housework and yardwork.

Be sure to download your Exercise Plan at **www.melioguide.com/exercise-plans** and have it in hand.

There are two major exercise sections in this chapter. The Active Level Exercises are categorized into Warm Up and Strength. As you progress through the chapter, the type of exercise (Warm Up, Strength) will be indicated at the bottom of each page.

The Cardiovascular, Flexibility, and Postural Exercises have been covered in earlier chapters. Please refer to these chapters for more detail.

The frequency and progression of the **Warm Up** and **Strength** exercises should be followed as described in your Exercise Plan. For the Strength exercises you will require dumbbells, an exercise mat or comfortable carpet to lie on, and a step. The equipment you will need can be found at most major outlet stores. If you feel any discomfort with any of the exercises, you should consult with a Physical Therapist before proceeding further.

Before you start, let me clarify what I mean in the Exercise Plan when I say "sets" and "reps." **Reps** is an abbreviation for repetitions. This is the number of repetitions you do before your muscles are too tired to do any more. Thus, if I ask you to do a set of ten repetitions, I want you to pick a weight that makes the exercise hard enough that by the tenth repetition the muscle you are targeting is very fatigued and you would have a hard time completing another repetition with good form. If the recommended second set indicates that you perform fewer repetitions than the first set, then you should choose a heavier weight or slow down your cadence.

Sets represent the number of times you redo the exercise. If I ask you to do two sets you should not do them back-to-back. The muscle being targeted needs time to recover – a full minute at the very least!

This doesn't mean you have to sit around and wait. Your recovery time can be used working another muscle group or working on your Balance exercises. I designed the exercise series so that you could do them one after another. This approach allows for an active recovery period. This saves you time and builds a cardiovascular component into your program.

Under the Strength Exercises I have listed the main muscles involved in executing the exercise as well as which part of your skeleton gets the most stimulation from the exercise. The three most frequent bone fracture areas (spine, hip, and wrist) are identified. The muscle groups and affected bones are listed under "Targets."

For example, while doing a squat, your muscles at the front of your thighs and your buttocks are the most active and your hip bones are loaded. Your spine gets loaded as you hold your chest forward, hold a weight or wear a weighted vest while doing your squat.

Use of Affirmations During the Warm Up Exercises

You should use personal affirmations as you go through your Warm Ups to start your session off on the right foot and get yourself into the right frame of mind. An affirmation is a positive personal thought. As you inhale, say to yourself "I am." As you exhale, choose an affirmation to take with you into your workout: "energized"... "balanced" ... "strong" .... "focussed". Now onto your first Warm Up Exercise.

WARM UP 1 – ENERGY TREE

STARTING POSITION:

» Stand tall.

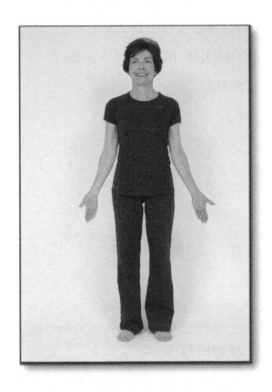

MOVEMENT:

» Inhale as you raise your arms overhead and lengthen the space between your pelvis and rib cage(imagine you're gathering energy from the sky).

» Exhale as you drop your shoulders away from your ears and then lower your hands down by your side.

» Repeat.

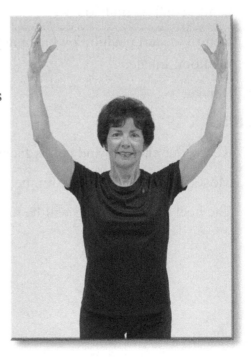

Active Warm Up Exercises

WARM UP 2 – CURTSEY

STARTING POSITION:

» Stand tall with palms together.

» Inhale.

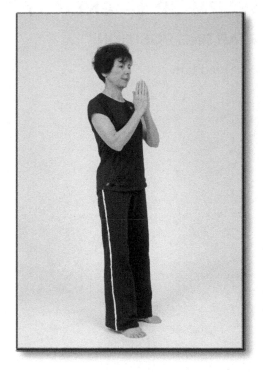

MOVEMENT:

» Exhale as you cross your left leg behind your right, gently bending both knees.

» Return to start position by pushing your front foot into the floor. Inhale.

» Repeat.

TIPS:

» Keep your chest up and pelvis facing forward.

» Most of the weight will be on the front leg.

» The heel of the back leg will be raised.

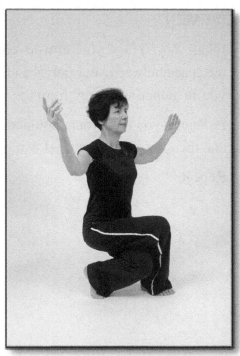

Active Warm Up Exercises

WARM UP 3 – MARCHING

STARTING POSITION:

» Stand tall.

MOVEMENT:

» March on the spot as you breathe in and out.

» Simultaneously swing your opposite arm towards the ceiling as you march.

» Raise your knees as high as you comfortably can. If you feel unstable you should do this between two chairs.

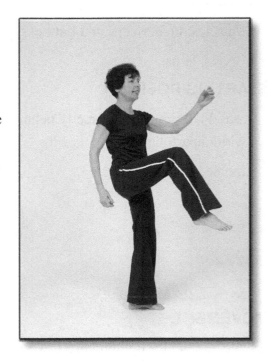

TIPS:

» Swinging your arms with a bent elbow will allow you to march at a quicker pace. This has good carryover for brisk walking.

Active Warm Up Exercises

CHAIR SQUATS

TARGETS:

» Muscles: Quadriceps and buttocks.

» Bones: Hips.

STARTING POSITION:

» Stand tall with chair directly behind you, feet shoulder width apart, hands on your hips.

» Inhale.

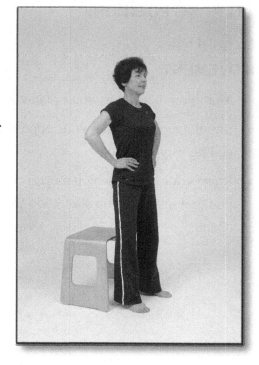

MOVEMENT:

Exhale and gently tighten your lower tummy as you:

» Sit back toward the chair behind you.

» Keep the middle of your knee pointing in the same direction as your second toe and your weight evenly distributed between your heel and forefoot.

» Eyes forward.

» Squat, only as far as you can, while maintaining proper posture and knee alignment.

» Repeat the movement until the set is completed.

TIPS:

» Stay in control of the movement the entire time. Go down as far as you can toward the chair without actually sitting on it.

» Squeeze your buttocks and push the floor away from you as you return to a standing position.

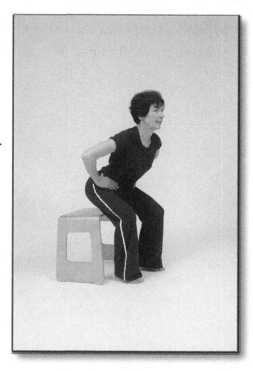

Active Strength Exercises

FLOOR M'S

TARGETS:

» Muscles: Neck extensors, spinal extensors, back, and shoulders.

» Bones: Spine.

STARTING POSITION:

» Lie face down with a pillow under your pelvis and rolled towel under your forehead.

» Arms rest at your side.

» Inhale.

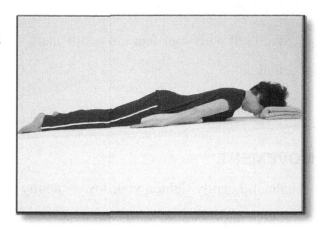

MOVEMENT:

Exhale and gently press the front of your pelvis into the pillow as you:

» Simultaneously, raise your head, chest, and arms off the floor while drawing your shoulder blades downward and together.

» Rotate your arms to open up your chest. Turn your palms away from you with your thumbs pointed toward the ceiling.

» Return to starting position and repeat until set is completed.

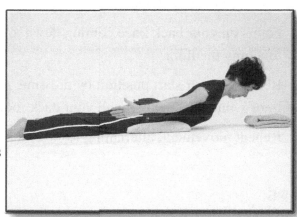

TIPS:

» Do not lift your chin away from your chest as you lift. Keep your gaze on the towel.

» Large-breasted women should use two pillows under their pelvis and a taller towel roll under their forehead.

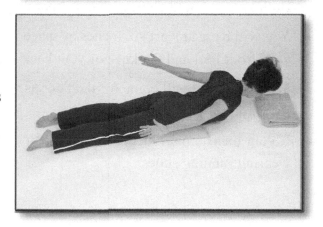

Active Strength Exercises

FORWARD LUNGE

TARGETS:

» Muscles: Hamstrings, buttocks, and quadriceps.

» Bones: Hips and spine.

STARTING POSITION:

» Stand tall with your feet hip width apart.

» Inhale.

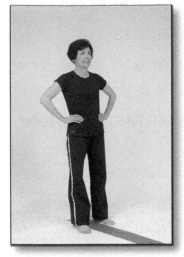

MOVEMENT:

Exhale and gently tighten your lower tummy as you:

» Take a large step forward.

» Lower your hips as you keep your head, shoulders, and hips in line over your back knee.

» Focus on your back knee coming down toward the floor, but not touching the floor.

» Return to your start position by pressing your front leg into the floor while pushing off with your back foot.

» Repeat movement, alternating legs, until set is completed.

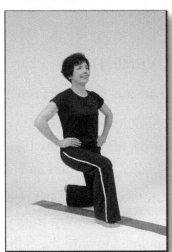

TIPS:

» Both knees should align with corresponding second toe.

» You will have at least six inches of space between your heel of your front foot and the knee of your back leg.

» Your back heel will come off the floor as you transfer your weight forward.

» If your toes do not like the pressure, you may try this exercise wearing running shoes.

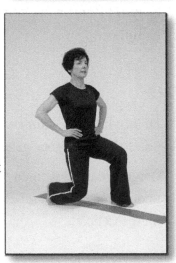

Active Strength Exercises

HORSE STANCE HORIZONTAL

TARGETS:

» Muscles: Deep back muscles.

» Bones: Spine and wrist.

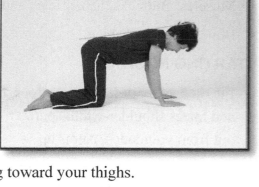

STARTING POSITION:

» Assume a four-point kneeling position.

» Keep your knees directly under your hips and your hands directly under your shoulders.

» Keep your elbows unlocked, with your elbows pointing toward your thighs.

» You should have a hand-width space in your low back. A yardstick along your spine would keep you in perfect alignment. Contact points will be your pelvis, mid-back, and back of head.

» With your spine kept in a neutral alignment position, take a deep diaphragmatic breath in allowing your belly to drop towards the floor.

MOVEMENT:

Exhale and gently tighten your lower tummy as you:

» Straighten your one arm level with your torso.

» Hold this position for up to five seconds.

» Repeat this pattern with your opposite arm, your left leg, and your right leg (one at a time!)

» Each individual lift corresponds to a single repetition on your Exercise Schedule.

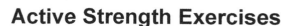

TIPS:

» If you are unable to tolerate resting on your wrist, you can do the exercise with your forearms on a small bench, with a small towel rolled under your palms (but not your fingers), or on your knuckles.

» You can place a yardstick along your spine to ensure perfect alignment.

» Throughout the exercise, keep your spine motionless.

» As your back gets stronger and you want more of a challenge, try raising your opposite arm and leg simultaneously. This is considered an "advanced" Horse Stance position and is worthwhile trying to master.

Active Strength Exercises

BRIDGING WITH WEIGHT ON PELVIS

TARGETS:

» Muscles: Buttocks, hamstrings, and back.

» Bones: Hips and spine.

STARTING POSITION:

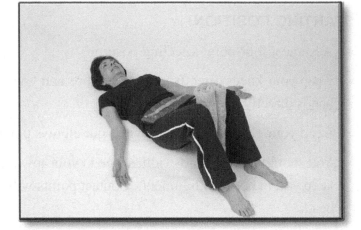

» Lie on back with feet flat on floor, feet and knees shoulder-width apart, arms out from your sides, palms up.

» Hold a rolled towel between your legs.

» Place a sand bag weight (two to five pounds) on your pelvis.

» Inhale.

MOVEMENT:

Exhale as you:

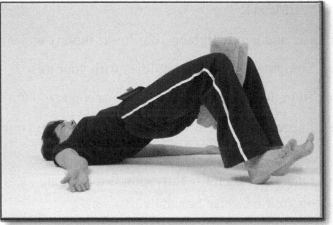

» Squeeze your buttocks and push down through your heels.

» Transfer your weight onto your shoulder blades as you lift your hips towards the ceiling.

» Raise your toes as you raise your hips, lowering your toes as you lower your hips.

» As you come down lengthen your spine as though your tail-bone is reaching towards your heels.

» Return in a controlled manner to starting position and repeat movement until set is completed.

TIP:

» You should feel this in your buttocks, back of your thighs, and muscles along your spine.

» Transfer your body weight to your heels and shoulder blades and not the back of your neck.

» Go high enough that you are bringing your hips into the line drawn between your hips and shoulders.

Active Strength Exercises

ROW WITH SUPPORT

TARGETS:

» Muscles: Upper back, buttocks, and hamstrings.

» Bones: Hips, spine, and wrist.

STARTING POSITION:

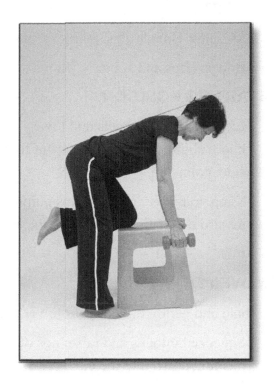

» Bend forward from your hips to bring one hand and knee on a padded chair or stool. Rest the weight on the chair.

» Your supporting leg should rest along side the chair/stool with your knee bent.

» Keep a slight inward arch in your low back.

» Grasp the dumbbell in your free hand and drop it straight down from your shoulder without locking your elbow.

» Inhale.

MOVEMENT:

Exhale and gently tighten your lower tummy as you:

» Pull your elbow to your side simultaneously drawing your shoulder blade towards your spine.

» Maintain your body position throughout move.

» Return to start position and repeat movement until set is completed.

» Switch sides and repeat.

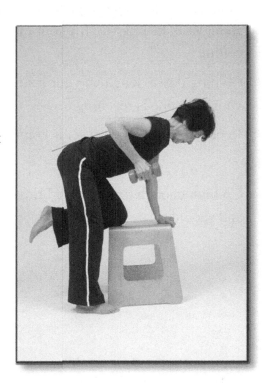

TIPS:

» Keep your supporting elbow unlocked.

» Keep your supporting knee unlocked.

» Stick your butt out to help you keep your spine properly aligned. (There should be a slight arch in your low back.)

Active Strength Exercises

HIP RAISE WITH FEET ON CHAIR

TARGETS:

» Muscles: Hamstrings, buttocks, and back.

» Bones: Hips and spine.

STARTING POSITION:

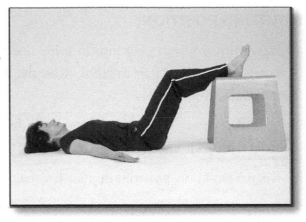

» Lie on back with heels and lower legs on chair, knees slightly bent and arms out from your side, palms up.

» Keep your feet and kneecaps pointed upwards toward the ceiling throughout the exercise.

» Inhale.

MOVEMENT:

Exhale and gently tighten your lower tummy as you:

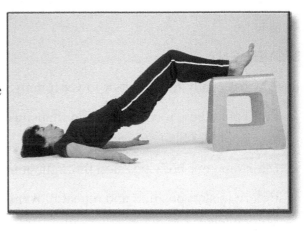

» Squeeze buttocks and raise hips off the ground pushing down into the chair.

» Transfer your weight to your heels and shoulder blades as you lift your hips toward the ceiling.

» Coming down, lengthen your spine as though your tail bone is reaching toward the chair.

» Repeat movement until set is completed.

TIP:

» Go high enough that you are bringing your hips into the line drawn between your hips, knees and shoulders.

Active Strength Exercises

SIDE LYING LEG LIFT WITH WEIGHT

TARGETS:

» Muscles: Abductors.

» Bones: Hips.

STARTING POSITION:

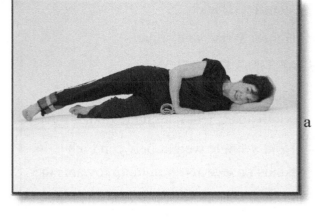
a

» Lie on your side against a wall with head, neck, back, hips, and top leg forming straight line with your body and your foot pulled towards your shin.

» Bottom leg should be comfortably bent.

» Your top hand should be on the floor in front of your belly button to help maintain your position.

» Rest your head on your bottom arm or a pillow. Inhale.

MOVEMENT:

Exhale and gently tighten your lower tummy as you:

» Keep your heel in contact with the wall and slowly lift your top leg.

» Turn your kneecap and foot slightly to the ceiling as you lift and lower your leg (not shown).

» Repeat the movement until your set is completed.

» Switch leg and repeat movement.

TIPS:

» If your hips are wider than your waist, place a small pillow or rolled towel in the space between your pelvis and rib cage.

» Your top heel should remain in contact with the wall throughout the exercise.

» The closer to the ankle the weight is placed the heavier it will feel.

» If you are unable to do the required number of repetitions with the weight at your ankle, start with it resting on your thigh above your knee and slide it down as you get stronger.

Active Strength Exercises

PULLOVERS FROM FLOOR

TARGETS:

» Muscles: Back.

» Bones: Wrists and spine.

STARTING POSITION:

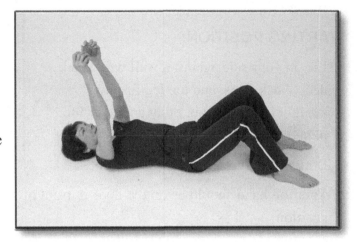

» Lie on your back, knees and feet hip-width apart, feet flat on the floor.

» Hold a single weight between both hands raise arms straight up towards the ceiling.

» Inhale.

MOVEMENT:

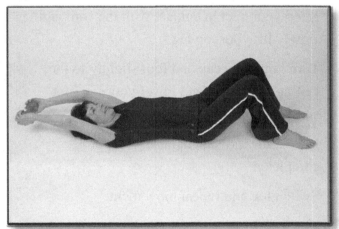

Exhale and gently tighten your lower tummy as you:

» Move the weight overhead until your upper arms are beside your ears.

» Slowly return the weight to the start position.

» Repeat movement until the set is completed.

TIPS:

» Your elbows should remain straight but not locked.

» This is a good time to consider wearing weight training gloves to maximize your grip.

Active Strength Exercises

STEP PUSH UP

TARGETS:

» Muscles: Chest, triceps, and abdominals.

» Bones: Wrists and spine.

STARTING POSITION:

» Use a stable surface – counter tops, steps, or stable stools work great.

» Place your hands one and one-half shoulder-width apart on the surface with your hands turned slightly towards each other

» Keep your head, shoulder, hips, and ankles in line.

» Inhale.

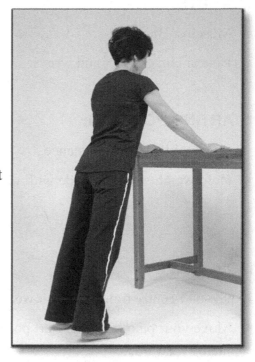

MOVEMENT:

Exhale and gently tighten your lower tummy as you:

» Lower your body towards the counter or step, bending your elbows away from you.

» Push away, straightening but not locking the elbows.

» Repeat movement until the set is completed.

TIPS:

» Keep your head, shoulders, hips, and ankles in line throughout the exercise.

» Let yourself rock forward onto the balls of your feet, lifting your heels.

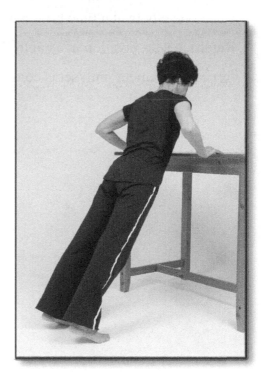

Active Strength Exercises

ALTERNATING BICEP CURL STANDING

TARGETS:

» Muscles: Biceps.

» Bones: Hips, spine, and wrists.

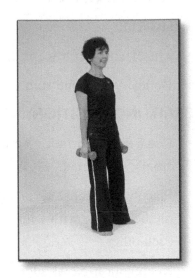

STARTING POSITION:

» Stand with an athletic stance.

» Hold weights by your side with your palms facing your thighs.

» Inhale.

MOVEMENT:

Exhale and gently tighten your lower tummy as you:

» Move your palm from its start position, facing thighs, to palm facing forward.

» Bend one elbow at a time bringing your hand to your shoulder.

» Return to start position in a controlled manner.

» Repeat movement until set is completed.

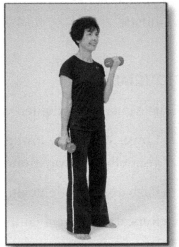

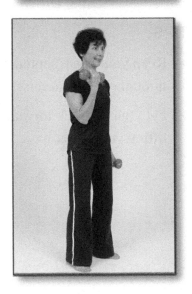

Active Strength Exercises

TRICEPS EXTENSION

TARGETS:

» Muscles: Triceps and shoulders.

» Bones: Wrists.

STARTING POSITION:

» Using good body mechanics, lie on your back, knees and feet hip-width apart.

» Hold weights in both hands with arms straight and (hand is in line with your forehead).

» Inhale.

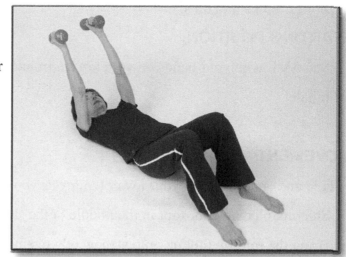

MOVEMENT:

Exhale and gently tighten your lower tummy as you:

» Bend arms at elbow, lowering weight until they almost reach the floor behind you (your hands should be on either side of head).

» Hold and return to start position.

» Repeat movement until set is completed.

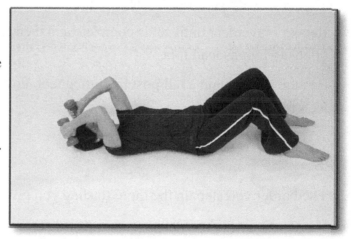

TIPS:

» Keep your upper arms steady through the bending and straightening of your elbow.

» Do not lock your elbows.

Active Strength Exercises

STEP UPS

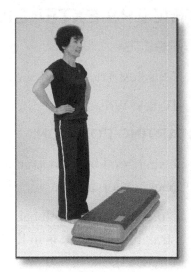

TARGETS:

» Muscles: Calves, quadriceps, and buttocks.

» Bones: Spine and hips.

STARTING POSITION:

» Stand tall with your hands on your hips in front of the step.

» Inhale.

MOVEMENT:

Exhale and gently tighten your lower tummy as you:

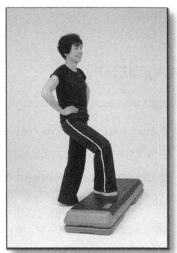

» Step up, placing your foot in the middle of the step.

» Bring the trailing foot up onto step, gently resting toe on the step and keeping your weight on your leading leg.

» Step back with your trailing leg leading.

» Repeat movement until set is complete and then repeat using opposite foot as lead foot.

» Be sure to maintain a tall posture throughout movement – do not lean forward.

TIPS:

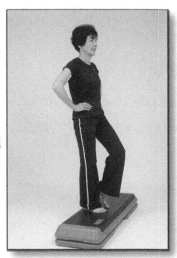

» The harder you step up the more loading you give your bones.

» Removing your shoes helps your bones absorb more of the force rather than the impact being taken through your shoes.

» You can use your stairs at home or sturdy bench.

» If you are not sure about how stable you will be, place your hand just above a chair placed near the step.

Active Strength Exercises

ABDOMINAL ACTIVATION WITH LEG DROP

TARGETS:

» Muscles: Transverse abdominus.

» Bones: Spine.

STARTING POSITION:

» Lie on your back, arms at your sides and hands palm up.

» Place a small rolled towel in the small of your back (roll should be the width and depth of your hand).

» Bend your knees and raise one leg then the other until both legs are off the floor as illustrated.

» Inhale.

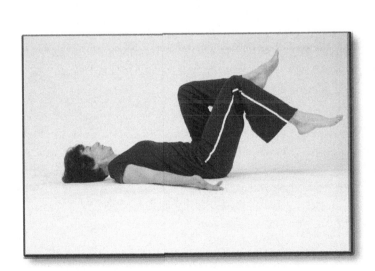

MOVEMENT:

Exhale and gently tighten your lower tummy as you:

» Alternate lower each leg and return to start position.

» Repeat movement until set is completed.

» When completed, drop one leg at a time back to the floor.

TIPS:

» If you are unable to keep your abdominals tight for the full set, then return to the start position, rest then when you are ready resume the set.

» The lower you drop your leg the greater the challenge.

Active Strength Exercises

12. Active Level Balance Exercises

Balance is a critical component of your exercise program. Balance becomes increasingly important as our bones age and become more fragile. We use our balance to keep us from falls that could lead to a fracture.

Increased balance allows you to be more independent and confident and can greatly affect the quality of your life. The more balanced you are when you perform day-to-day activities, the more likely you are to be active in life.

The balance exercises in this chapter have been developed for people who are either Low, Moderate, or High fracture risk.

These balance exercises will make you more stable and will have a direct impact on reducing your fracture risk. With practice, your balance will improve. Follow these instructions when you are performing your balance training:

» Choose among the exercises listed that challenge you.

» Make sure that you can hold your position for at least 10 seconds.

» Mix up the exercises from week to week for variety.

» Do a total of 3 to 5 minutes of balance training each session.

» Keep safety in mind by practicing your balance exercises in a safe location, such as a corner of a room with a sturdy chair in front of you for support.

» Maintain an athletic stance as discussed in Chapter 4.

WEIGHT TRANSFERS

» Take a step forward.

» Without moving your feet, transfer your weight forward and then back between your feet.

» Repeat 6 times.

» Switch foot positions.

» Repeat 6 times.

STEPPING FORWARD AND BACKWARD

» Take a step forward and transfer all your weight so that you are standing only on your front foot.

» Hold for 5 seconds.

» Step backward.

» Transfer all your weight so that you are standing only on your back foot.

» Repeat the motion 6 times.

» Repeat, leading with the other side.

WALKING THE LINE

This exercise is best done in a hallway where you can reach for support from the wall (if required) and can gauge your walk.

» Keep your hands available for balance.

» Walk as though you were on a tight rope. Step forward 10 steps.

» Progressively narrow the distance between your feet until you are walking heel to toe.

Active Balance Exercises

WALKING AS YOU LOOK AWAY

VERSION 1

» Slowly turn your head and eyes to the left and right as you walk straight ahead 10 steps.

VERSION 2

» Slowly tilt your head and eyes toward the ceiling and the floor as you walk straight ahead 10 steps.

VERSION 3

» Gradually try turning your head faster and further.

VERSION 4

» Walk as you read a newspaper.

TAKING A TURN

» Take a few steps; quickly turn 90 degrees, place your feet together and stop.

» Take a few steps, turn 180 degrees and stop.

» Practice turning in both directions. Repeat each turn 5 times.

PHYSIO BALL BALANCE EXERCISES

Please refer to the section Equipment Recommendations – Burst-Resistant Physio Ball in Chapter 1 for the correct type and size of Physio Ball. You should also review "Safely Using a Physio Ball" in Chapter 4 if you are unfamiliar with using a Physio Ball or if it has been a long time since you last were on one.

Try these moves on your Physio Ball:

» Sit over the center of the ball with your thighs supported on the ball.

» Shift your hips side to side.

» Shift your hips to one side and lift the opposite leg off the floor.

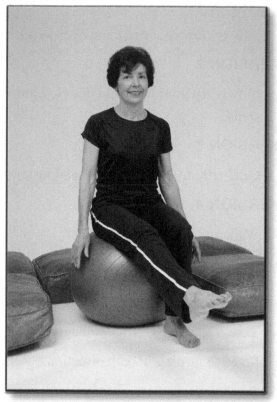

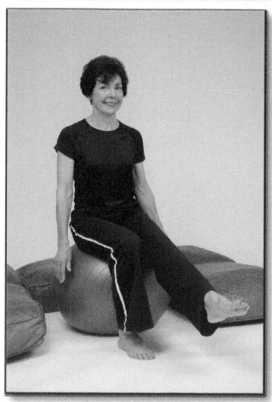

Active Balance Exercises

13. Athletic Level Strength Exercises

By now you should have read and completed the foundation chapters in this guide. You should be comfortable with your bone and body basics (Chapter 3), know the key exercise safety tips (Chapter 4), understand which exercises and poses you should avoid and why (Chapter 5), have optimized your posture (Chapter 6), have checked your flexibility (Chapter 7), and have selected the cardiovascular exercises are right for you (Chapter 8).

You should have determined your appropriate exercise level. Your activity level will be either Beginner, Active, Athletic, or Elite, and your fracture risk will be either Low, Moderate, or High (see Chapter 2).

Since you are reading the Athletic Level Exercise chapter, I am assuming that you have selected the Athletic Level. The Athletic Level Exercise program is designed for people who are either at a low or moderate fracture risk, and who have been involved in a regular exercise program (3 to 4 sessions per week). You have used or are not intimidated using an exercise/ Physio ball in your routine. You are involved in light sports such as golf, bowling, curling, or swimming.

Be sure to download your Exercise Plan at **www.melioguide.com/exercise-plans** and have it in hand.

There are two major exercise sections in this chapter. The Athletic Level Exercises are categorized into Warm Up and Strength. As you progress through the chapter, the type of exercise (Warm Up, Strength) will be indicated at the bottom of each page.

The Cardiovascular, Flexibility, and Postural Exercises have been covered in earlier chapters. Please refer to these chapters for more detail.

The frequency and progression of the **Warm Up** and **Strength** exercises should be followed as described in your Exercise Plan. For the Strength exercises you will require dumbbells, an exercise mat or comfortable carpet to lie on and a burst resistant exercise ball. The equipment you will need can be found at most major outlet stores. If you feel any discomfort with any of the exercises, you should consult with a Physical Therapist before proceeding further.

Before you start, let me clarify what I mean in the Exercise Plan when I say "sets" and "reps." **Reps** is an abbreviation for repetitions. This is the number of repetitions you do before your muscles are too tired to do any more. Thus, if I ask you to do a set of ten repetitions, I want you to pick a weight that makes the exercise hard enough that by the tenth repetition the muscle you are targeting is very fatigued and you would have a hard time completing another repetition with good form. If the recommended second set indicates that you perform fewer repetitions than the first set, then you should choose a heavier weight or slow down your cadence.

Sets represent the number of times you redo the exercise. If I ask you to do two sets you should not do them back-to-back. The muscle being targeted needs time to recover – a full minute at the very least!

This doesn't mean you have to sit around and wait. Your recovery time can be used working another muscle group or working on your Balance exercises. I designed the exercise series so that you could do them one after another. This approach allows for an active recovery period. This saves you time and builds a cardiovascular component into your program.

Under the Strength Exercises I have listed the prime or main muscles involved in executing the exercise as well as which part of your skeleton gets the most stimulation from the exercise. The three most frequent bone fracture areas (spine, hip, and wrist) are identified. The muscle groups and affected bones are listed under "Targets."

For example, while doing a squat, your muscles at the front of your thighs and your buttocks are the most active and your hip bones are loaded. Your spine gets loaded as you hold your chest forward, hold a weight, or wear a weighted vest while doing your squat.

Use of Affirmations During the Warm Up Exercises

You should use personal affirmations as you go through your Warm Ups to start your session off on the right foot and get yourself into the right frame of mind. An affirmation is a positive personal thought. As you inhale, say to yourself "I am." As you exhale, choose an affirmation to take with you into your workout: "energized"… "balanced" ... "strong" .... "focussed". Now onto your first Warm Up Exercise.

WARM UP 1 – LATERAL LUNGE

STARTING POSITION:

» Stand tall with your feet shoulder width apart.

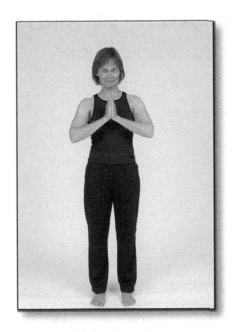

MOVEMENT:

» Take a large step out to the side as you transfer your weight to your right forward foot and heel.

» Keep your feet pointing forward and flat on the floor.

» Sit back behind your right heel and keep your back long, eyes forward, and chest open.

» Straighten your left leg but do not lock your left knee.

» Return to the standing position and repeat on the other side.

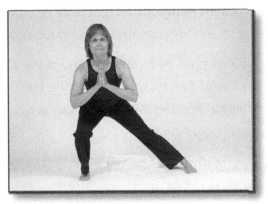

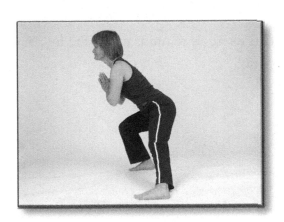

Athletic Warm Up Exercises

WARM UP 2 – BIRD NOD

STARTING POSITION:

» Stand tall, palms together.

» Inhale.

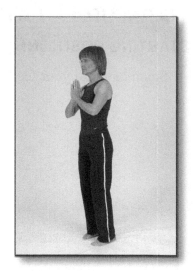

MOVEMENT:

Exhale and gently tighten your lower tummy as you:

» Transfer all your weight onto one leg, keeping your knee bent at a twenty degree angle, and raise your arms out to your side.

» Keep your body straight and pivot around your supporting hip joint as you raise your free leg back; simultaneously lower your trunk.

» Alternate feet until your set is done.

» Go down only as far as you are comfortable and able to keep your hips level.

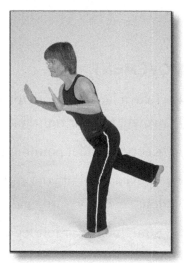

This exercise reminds me of the toy "nodding birds" – hence the name!

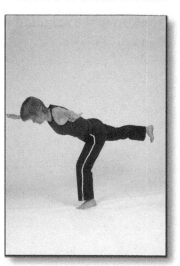

Athletic Warm Up Exercises

WARM UP 3 – LUNGE STEPS

STARTING POSITION:

» Place both hands in front of you on a 12 inch stable step.

» Place one foot back and the other forward close to the step and directly below the front knee.

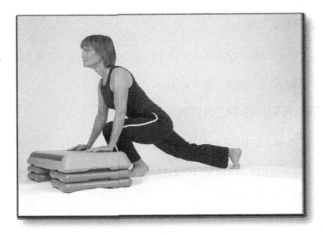

MOVEMENT:

» Press on the step with both hands and maintain the pressure.

» While maintaining your press position on the step, explosively move the back leg to the forward position and the forward foot to the back position in a lunge like fashion.

» Repeat the lunge.

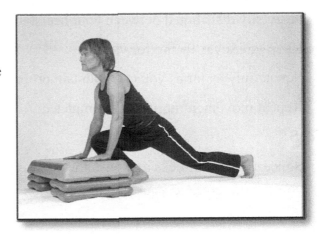

TIP

» Be sure you keep your back straight as you perform this exercise.

Athletic Warm Up Exercises

SQUATS WITH WEIGHTS

TARGETS:

» Muscles: Quadriceps, buttocks, and back extensors.

» Bones: Hips and spine.

STARTING POSITION:

» Stand with feet shoulder width apart.

» Weights should be held in both hands and resting on your shoulders.

» Inhale.

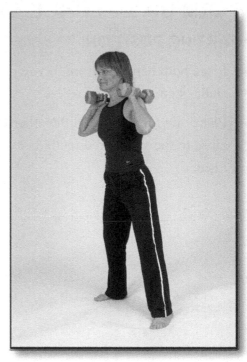

MOVEMENT:

Exhale and gently tighten your lower tummy as you:

» Squat, keep the middle of your knee pointing in the same direction as your second toe; your weight should be evenly distributed between your heel and forefoot.

» Keep your eyes facing forward.

» Squat, only as far as you can maintain proper alignment.

» Repeat movement until set is completed.

TIPS:

» Squeeze your buttocks and push the floor away from you as you return to your standing position.

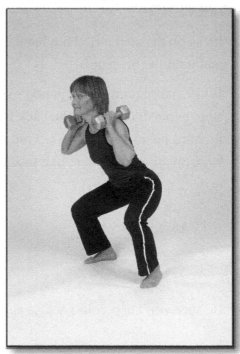

Athletic Strength Exercises

BALL T'S

TARGETS:

» Muscles: Neck extensors, spinal extensors, back, shoulders, and buttocks.

» Bones: Spine.

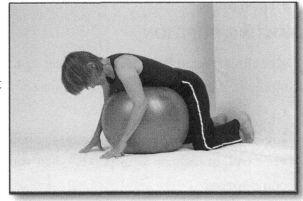

STARTING POSITION:

» Kneeling behind ball, place your feet against stable surface, hip-width apart with knees bent (a wall works well for support).

» Lie over the top of the ball (mount the ball so your weight rests on your pelvis when you come forward).

» Arms should be resting in front of the ball.

» Inhale.

MOVEMENT:

Exhale and gently tighten your lower tummy as you:

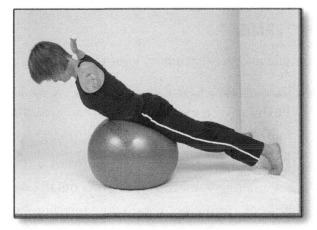

» Push forward extending your torso over the ball.

» Pull your shoulder blades downward and together as you bring your arms out to create a "T" formation. Lead with your thumbs and keep your elbows unlocked.

» Keep your head and spine in line.

TIP:

» Your toes should remain on the floor and your heels against the stable surface. This will prepare you for doing the exercise without support.

» Do not lift your chin away from your chest as you raise your body and arms.

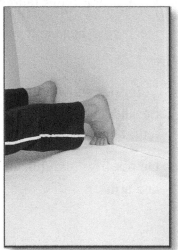

Athletic Strength Exercises

BALL M'S

TARGETS:

» Muscles: Neck extensors, spinal extensors, back, shoulders, and buttocks.

» Bones: Spine.

STARTING POSITION:

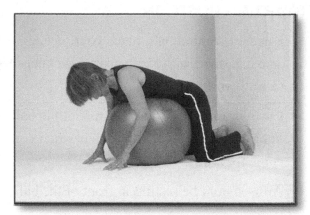

» Kneeling behind ball, place your feet against stable surface hip-width apart with knees bent (a wall works well for support).

» Lie over the top of the ball (mount the ball so your weight rests on your pelvis when you come forward).

» Arms should be resting in front of the ball.

» Inhale.

MOVEMENT:

Exhale and gently tighten your lower tummy as you:

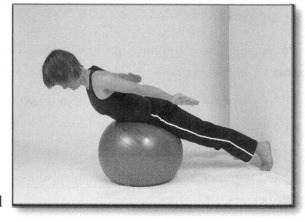

» Push forward extending your torso over the ball.

» Pull your shoulder blades downward and together as you bring your arms out to create an "M" formation. Lead with your thumbs and keep your elbows unlocked.

» Keep your head and spine in line.

TIP:

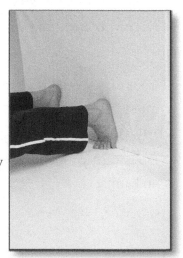

» Your toes should remain on the floor and your heels against the stable surface. This will prepare you for doing the exercise without support.

» Do not lift your chin away from your chest as you raise your body and arms.

Athletic Strength Exercises

BALL Y'S

TARGETS:

» Muscles: Neck extensors, spinal extensors, back, shoulders, and buttocks.

» Bones: Spine.

STARTING POSITION:

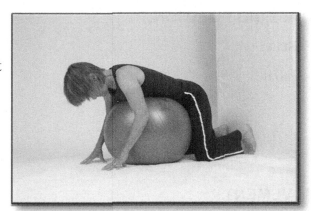

» Kneeling behind ball, place your feet against stable surface hip-width apart with knees bent (a wall works well for support).

» Lie over the top of the ball (mount the ball so your weight rests on your pelvis when you come forward).

» Arms should be resting in front of the ball.

» Inhale.

MOVEMENT:

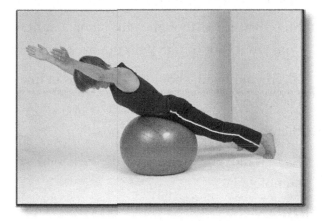

Exhale and gently tighten your lower tummy as you:

» Push forward extending your torso over the ball.

» Pull your shoulder blades downward and together as you bring your arms out to create a "Y" formation. Lead with your thumbs and keep your elbows unlocked.

» Keep your head and spine in line.

TIP:

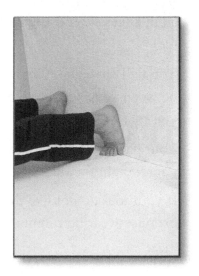

» Your toes should remain on the floor and your heels against the stable surface. This will prepare you for doing the exercise without support.

» Do not lift your chin away from your chest as you raise your body and arms.

Athletic Strength Exercises

LUNGE IN LINE

TARGETS:

» Muscles: Hamstrings, buttocks, and quadriceps.

» Bones: Hips and spine.

STARTING POSITION:

» Stand tall.

» Inhale.

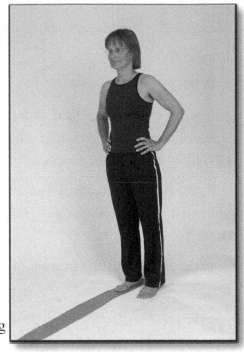

MOVEMENT:

Exhale and gently tighten your lower tummy as you:

» Step forward as though walking on a tight rope (keeping your front foot in line with the back foot and knee)

» Keep your head, shoulders, and hips in line over your back knee.

» Step back returning to start position.

» Repeat movement, alternating legs, until set is completed.

TIPS:

» Both knees should align with corresponding second toe.

» You will have about four to six inches of space between your heel of your front foot and the knee of your back leg.

» Your back heel will come off the floor as you transfer your weight forward.

» If your toes do not like the pressure, you may try this exercise wearing running shoes.

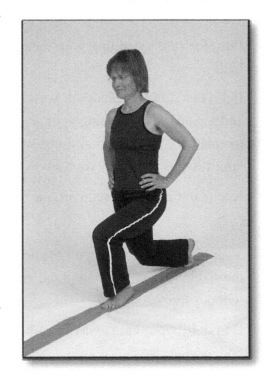

Athletic Strength Exercises

OVERHEAD LIFT

TARGETS:

» Muscles: Shoulders, quadriceps, and buttocks.

» Bones: Hips, spine, and wrist.

STARTING POSITION:

» Stand with one foot on an elevated step and hold weights while keeping your hips and chest facing forward.

» Inhale.

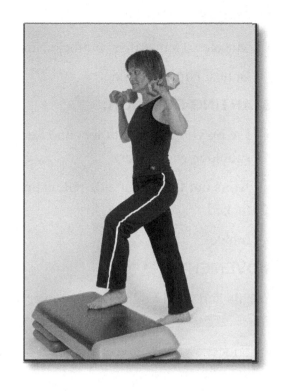

MOVEMENT:

Exhale and gently tighten your lower tummy as you:

» Raise the weights overhead.

» Hold and return weights to start position.

» Repeat movement until set is completed.

TIP:

» Do not lock elbows or your supporting knee.

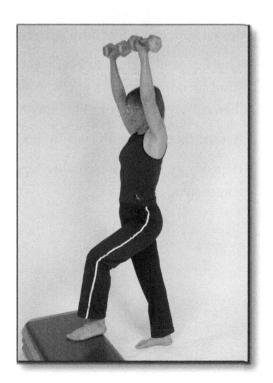

Athletic Strength Exercises

BRIDGING – UP 2 / DOWN 1

TARGETS:

» Muscles: Hamstrings, buttocks, and back.

» Bones: Hips and spine.

STARTING POSITION:

» Lie on your back with feet and knees shoulder-width apart.

» Arms out from your side palms up, shoulders tucked.

» Inhale.

MOVEMENT:

Exhale and gently tighten your lower tummy as you:

» Squeeze your buttocks and push both heels into the ground.

» Raise your hips to the height of a straight line drawn between your shoulders and knees.

» Transfer your weight to one heel and straighten the opposite leg from the knee and then slowly lower your buttocks back to floor.

» Return foot to floor in starting position.

» Repeat movement, alternating legs, until set is completed.

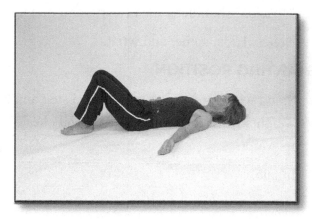

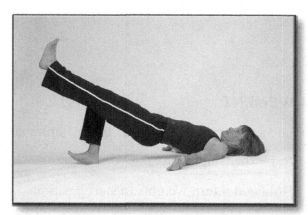

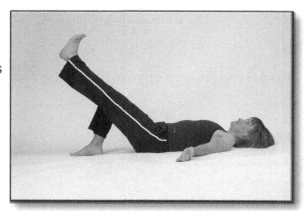

Athletic Strength Exercises

ROW – HAND SUPPORT ONLY

TARGETS:

» Muscles: Upper back, buttocks, and hamstrings.

» Bones: Hips, spine, and wrist.

STARTING POSITION:

Holding a dumbbell weight:

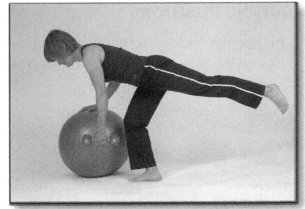

» Bend forward from your hips and place one hand on a supporting surface (a ball or chair works well).

» Raise your leg on the same side as the dumbbell weight and keep your pelvis level.

» Lower your arm holding the weight straight down from your shoulder without locking your elbow.

» Inhale.

MOVEMENT:

Exhale and gently tighten your lower tummy as you:

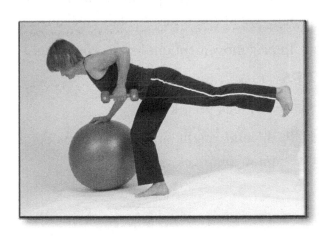

» Pull your elbow to your side simultaneously drawing your shoulder blade towards your spine.

» Maintain your body position throughout the exercise.

» Repeat movement until set is completed.

» Switch supporting legs when you switch sides and repeat.

Athletic Strength Exercises

HIP RAISES – FEET ON BALL

TARGETS:

» Muscles: Buttocks, back, and hamstrings.

» Bones: Hips and spine.

STARTING POSITION:

» Lie on your back with your heels and lower legs on the ball, knees slightly bent and arms out from your side, palms up.

» Inhale.

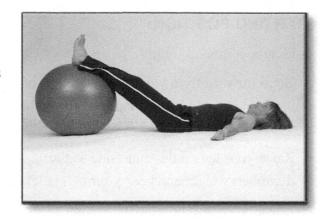

MOVEMENT:

Exhale and gently tighten your lower tummy as you:

» Squeeze buttocks and raise hips off the ground until your ankles, hips, and shoulders are all in line – hold and return to start position.

» Repeat movement until set is completed.

TIPS:

» Do not lock your knees.

» Push your weight through your shoulder blades and not your neck.

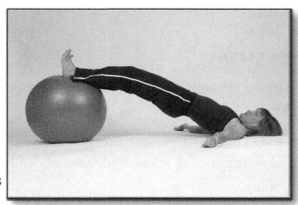

Athletic Strength Exercises

BAND WALKS

TARGETS:

» Muscles: Hip abductors and back.

» Bones: Hips and spine.

STARTING POSITION:

» Place a band around both ankles and widen feet until there is tension on the band.

» Stand with your feet slightly pigeon-toed.

» Inhale.

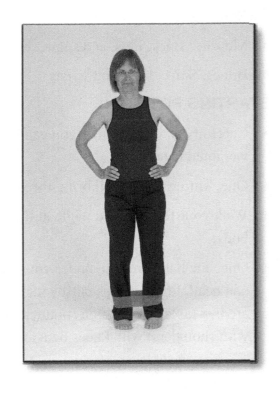

MOVEMENT:

Exhale and gently tighten your lower tummy as you:

» Lead with your heel. Step as wide as you can.

» Keep your torso over your supporting leg as you step.

» Catch up with a half step, always keeping a little tension on the band.

» If you are in a small space, take several steps to the right and two steps to the left until your set is complete.

» Repeat movement until set is completed. Finish your set by stepping toward your right.

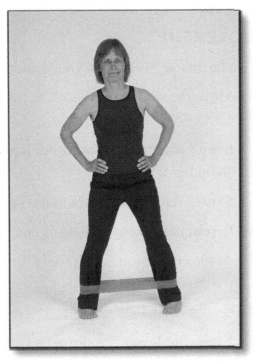

Athletic Strength Exercises

PULLOVER ON BALL (WITH SINGLE WEIGHT)

TARGETS:

» Muscles: Back, hips, and spinal extensors.

» Bones: Spine, hips, and wrists.

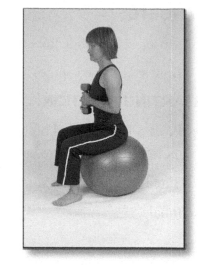

STARTING POSITION:

» Carefully sit on the ball – you can stabilize it by resting your weighted hand on it.

» Once sitting on the ball bring the weight against your chest.

» Walk your feet forward while at the same time lowering your body.

» Once the ball is resting under your upper shoulder blades and head, lift your hips until your torso and thighs are in a table-top position (buttocks and thighs in line with shoulders) with knees bent at right angles.

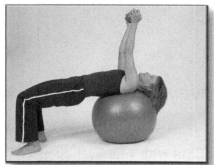

» Raise the weight towards the ceiling, holding it between both hands.

» Inhale.

MOVEMENT:

Exhale and gently tighten your lower tummy as you:

» Move the weight overhead until your arms are beside your ears.

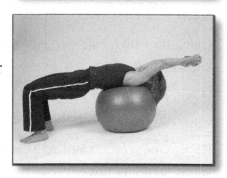

» Keep your buttocks squeezed. Keep hips in line with your shoulders and knees.

» Slowly return the weight to the start position.

» Repeat movement until set is completed.

» At the end of your set, lower your hips before you lower your weight to the ground.

TIP:

» Keep your lower ribs down as you raise your arms behind you.

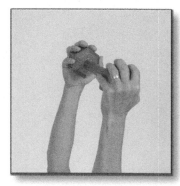

Athletic Strength Exercises

FLOOR PUSHUP

TARGETS:

» Muscles: Chest, triceps, and abdominals.

» Bones: Wrists, spine, and hips.

STARTING POSITION:

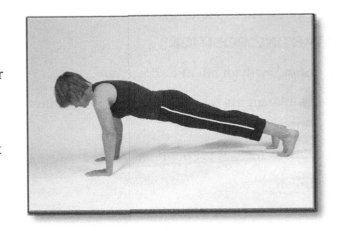

» Place your hands one and one-half shoulder width apart on the floor with your hands turned slightly toward each other.

» Step back onto the balls of your feet so that your body is in a straight line.

» Inhale.

MOVEMENT:

Exhale and gently tighten your lower tummy as you:

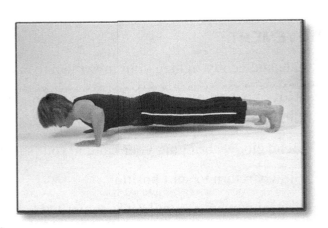

» Lower your body toward floor, bending your elbows until your upper arms are parallel to the floor.

» Push your body up away from floor by straightening your arms.

» Keep your head and spine in line.

» Repeat movement until your set is completed.

TIP:

» Keep your hips in a straight line drawn between your shoulders, hips, and ankles.

Athletic Strength Exercises

SINGLE LEG BICEPS CURL

TARGETS:

» Muscles: Biceps, buttocks, and quadriceps.

» Bones: Hips, spine, and wrists.

STARTING POSITION:

» Stand with an athletic stance.

» Hold weights by your side with your palms facing your thighs.

» Raise one foot off the floor.

» Inhale.

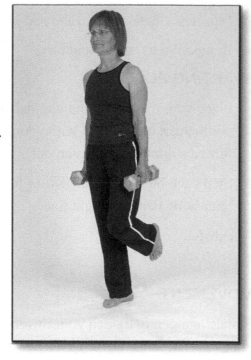

MOVEMENT:

Exhale and gently tighten your lower tummy as you:

» Move your palms from their start position, facing thighs, to palms facing forward

» Bend elbows bringing your hand to your shoulders.

» Slowly return to start position.

» Repeat movement until set is completed.

» Do half your set on each foot.

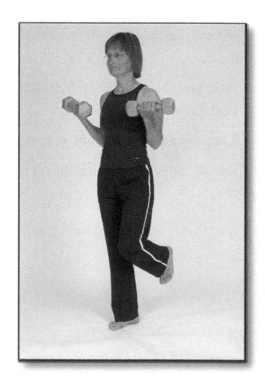

Athletic Strength Exercises

TRICEP EXTENSIONS ON BALL

TARGETS:

» Muscles: Triceps, shoulders, buttocks, and hamstrings.

» Bones: Wrists, hips, and spine.

STARTING POSITION:

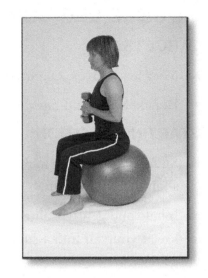

» Carefully sit on the ball – you can stabilize it by resting a weighted hand on it.

» Once sitting on the ball bring the weight against your chest.

» Walk your feet forward while at the same time lowering your body.

» Once the ball is resting under your upper shoulder blades and head, lift your hips until your torso and thighs are in a table-top position (buttocks and thighs in line with shoulders) with knees bent at right angles.

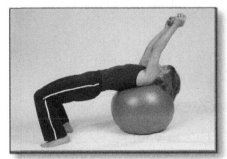

» Arms are straight and raised slightly higher than shoulder height (hands are in line with your eyes).

» Inhale.

MOVEMENT:

Exhale and gently tighten your lower tummy as you:

» Bend arms at elbow, lowering the weight until it reaches the ball behind you.

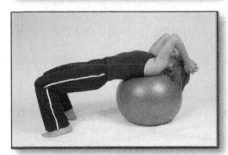

» Hold and return to start position.

» Repeat movement until set is completed.

TIPS:

» Keep your upper arms still through the bending and straightening of your elbow.

» Do not lock your elbows.

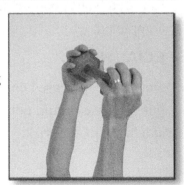

» Lower your hips before you lower the weight to the ground.

» Walk yourself back to a seated position.

Athletic Strength Exercises

DOUBLE LEG JUMP DOWN

TARGETS:

» Muscles: Calves, quadriceps, and buttocks.

» Bones: Spine and hips.

STARTING POSITION:

» Stand on a 6- to 10-inch high-step with your feet shoulder width apart.

» Inhale and gently tighten your lower tummy as you lower yourself into a squat.

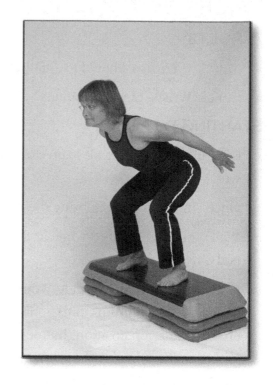

MOVEMENT:

Exhale as you:

» Explosively straighten knees to come out of the squat, jumping forward off the step.

» Land with your feet hip width apart and knees tracking over your second toe.

» Absorb the jump by allowing your knees to bend as you land.

» Return to start position and repeat until set is completed.

SPECIAL NOTE:

» Due to the increased compression forces upon landing, this exercise should not be done by individuals who are at a high fracture risk.

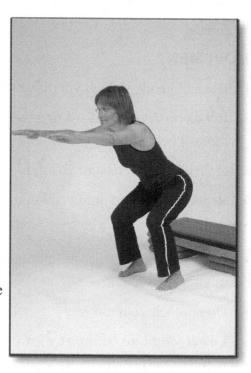

Athletic Strength Exercises

ABDOMINAL ACTIVATION WITH DROP 90/90

TARGETS:

» Muscles: Transverse abdominus.

» Bones: Spine.

STARTING POSITION:

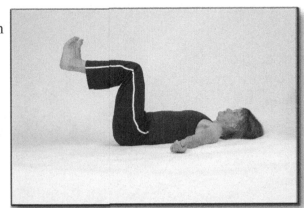

» Lie on floor with knees bent and feet hip width apart.

» Place a small rolled towel in the small of your back (roll should be the width and depth of your hand).

» Knees bent, raise one leg then the other until both legs are off the floor to 90 degrees.

» Inhale.

MOVEMENT:

Exhale and gently tighten your lower tummy as you:

» Alternately lower each leg and return to start position.

» The goal is not to allow your lower back to lift off your hand (or the towel).

» Return foot to start position and repeat movement until set is complete; repeat using alternate foot.

TIPS:

» If you are unable to keep your abdominals tight for the full set, return to the start position and take a short rest between leg lifts.

» The lower you drop your leg the greater the challenge.

» Wearing shoes adds an extra weight and so you may wish to start this exercise without shoes.

Athletic Strength Exercises

14. Athletic Level Balance Exercises

Balance is a critical component of your exercise program. Balance becomes increasingly important as our bones age and become more fragile. We use our balance to keep us from falls that could lead to a fracture.

Increased balance allows you to be more independent and confident and can greatly affect the quality of your life. The more balanced you are when you perform day-to-day activities, the more likely you are to be active in life.

The balance exercises in this chapter have been developed for people who are either Low or Moderate fracture risk. If you have a high fracture risk, please refer back to the Beginner or Active Level balance exercises (in Chapters 10 and 12).

The balance exercises will make you more stable and will have a direct impact on reducing your fracture risk. With practice, your balance will improve. Follow these instructions when you are performing your balance training:

» Choose among the exercises listed that challenge you.

» Make sure that you can hold your position for at least 10 seconds.

» Mix up the exercises from week to week for variety.

» Do a total of 3 to 5 minutes of balance training each session.

» Keep safety in mind by practicing your balance exercises in a safe location, such as a corner of a room with a sturdy chair in front of you for support.

» Maintain an athletic stance as discussed in Chapter 4.

FOUR POINT BALANCE ON BALL

The following exercise should be done using the correct sized ball as outlined in Chapter 2. Please review "Safely Using a Physio Ball" in Chapter 4.

STARTING POSITION:

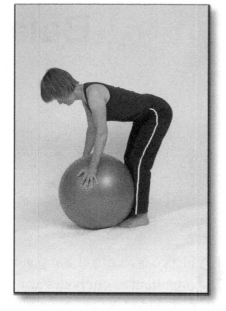

» Stand with your feet shoulder width apart and roll the ball against your shins.

» Place both hands on the ball directly under your shoulders.

MOVEMENT:

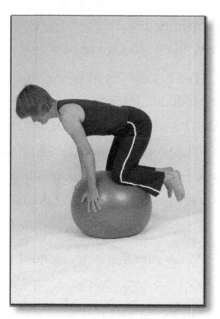

» Slowly roll ball forward by pushing off with your feet in a slow, controlled motion.

» Allow your shins to follow the motion of the ball until your knees are over the ball and your hands are on the front part of the ball.

» Back remains straight throughout the motion.

» Hold for up to 30 seconds.

Athletic Balance Exercises

THREE POINT BALANCE ON BALL

The following exercise should be done using the correct sized ball as outlined in Chapter 2. Please review "Safely Using a Physio Ball" in Chapter 4.

STARTING POSITION:

» Stand with your feet shoulder width apart and roll the ball against your shins.

» Place both hands on the ball directly under your shoulders.

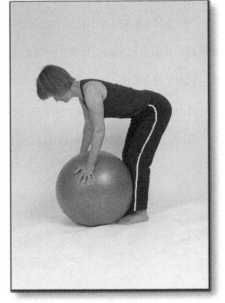

MOVEMENT:

» Slowly roll ball forward by pushing off with your feet in a slow, controlled motion.

» Allow your shins to follow the motion of the ball until your knees are over the ball and your hands are on the front part of the ball.

» Wiggle one hand to the midpoint location between both hands.

» Lift one arm while maintaining balance on ball

» Do both sides, holding for up to 10 seconds on each side.

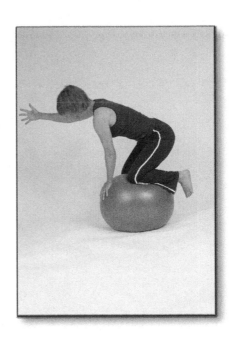

Athletic Balance Exercises

ON THE LINE

Stand on ½ foam roller with flat side down:

» Cross your arms over your chest.

» Step forward with your feet several inches apart.

» Hold for up to 20 seconds.

» Repeat with the other leg forward.

Next turn the ½ foam roller over so that the flat side is up:

» Repeat the pattern listed above.

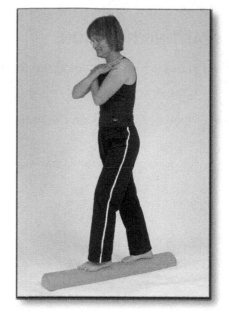

Athletic Balance Exercises

HEEL TO TOE

Stand on ½ foam roller with flat side down:

» Cross your arms over your chest.

» Now bring your feet closer together so that your heel of your forward foot is touching the toes on the back foot.

» Repeat for up to 20 seconds.

» Repeat with the other leg forward.

Next turn the ½ foam roller over so that the flat side is up:

» Repeat the pattern listed above.

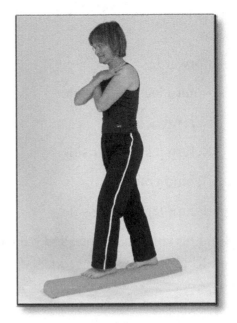

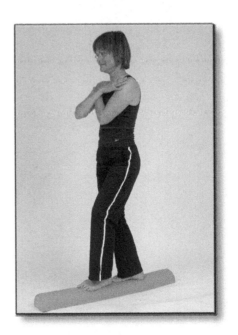

Athletic Balance Exercises

SINGLE LEG STANCE WITH MOVEMENT

Stand with one foot on the ½ foam roller or thick foam mat. Move the opposite leg in a slow controlled manner in the sequential order below:

» Forward.

» Return leg to your side.

» Sideways.

» Return leg to your side.

» Behind you.

» Return leg to your side.

Build up your endurance and balance to the point where you can comfortably repeat the sequence 6 times on each leg.

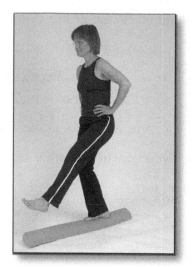

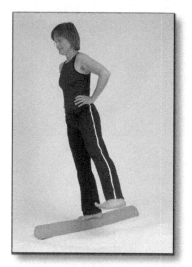

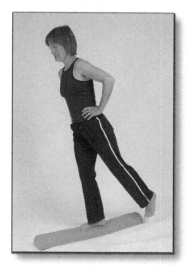

Athletic Balance Exercises

SINGLE LEG REACHES

» Arrange a set of cones or plastic pop bottles in a semicircle (approximately 6-foot or 2-metre diameter).

» Stand in the center of the cones and reach out to touch the cones with a single leg.

» Return to a full standing position on one leg between reaches.

» Repeat on opposite leg.

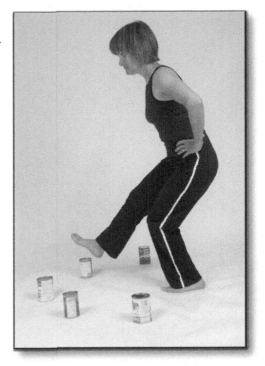

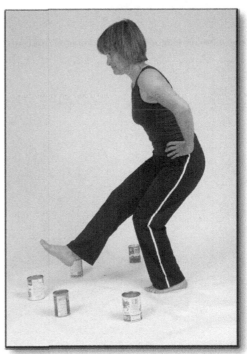

Athletic Balance Exercises

15. Elite Level Strength Exercises

By now you should have read and completed the foundation chapters in this guide. You should be comfortable with your bone and body basics (Chapter 3), know the key exercise safety tips (Chapter 4), understand which exercises and poses you should avoid and why (Chapter 5), have optimized your posture (Chapter 6), have checked your flexibility (Chapter 7), and have selected the cardiovascular exercises are right for you (Chapter 8).

You should have determined your appropriate Exercise level. Your activity level will be either Beginner, Active, Athletic, or Elite and your fracture risk will be either Low, Moderate, or High (see Chapter 2).

Since you are reading the Elite Level Exercise chapter, I am assuming that you have selected the Elite Level. The Elite Level Exercise program is designed for people who are at a low fracture risk, and have been involved in a frequent exercise program (4 to 7 times per week) that involves strength training for the past year and have used an exercise/Physio ball as part of their routine. If you have a high fracture risk (as indicated by your bone mineral density test), please refer back to the Beginner or Active Level programs.

Be sure to download your Exercise Plan at **www.melioguide.com/exercise-plans** and have it in hand.

There are two major exercise sections in this chapter. The Elite Level Exercises are categorized into Warm Up and Strength. As you progress through the chapter, the type of exercise (Warm Up, Strength) will be indicated at the bottom of each page.

The Cardiovascular, Flexibility, and Postural Exercises have been covered in earlier chapters. Please refer to these chapters for more detail.

The frequency and progression of the **Warm Up** and **Strength** exercises should be followed as described in your Exercise Plan. For the Strength exercises you will require dumbbells, an exercise mat or comfortable carpet to lie on, and a burst-resistant exercise ball. The equipment you will need can be found at most major outlet stores. If you feel any discomfort with any of the exercises, you should consult with a Physical Therapist before proceeding further.

Before you start, let me clarify what I mean in the Exercise Plan when I say "sets" and "reps." **Reps** is an abbreviation for repetitions. This is the number of repetitions you do before your muscles are too tired to do any more. Thus, if I ask you to do a set of ten repetitions, I want you to pick a weight that makes the exercise hard enough that by the tenth repetition the muscle you are targeting is very fatigued and you would have a hard time completing another repetition with good form. If the recommended second set indicates that you perform fewer repetitions than the first set, then you should choose a heavier weight or slow down your cadence.

Sets represent the number of times you redo the exercise. If I ask you to do two sets you should not do them back-to-back. The muscle being targeted needs time to recover – a full minute at the very least!

This doesn't mean you have to sit around and wait. Your recovery time can be used working another muscle group or working on your Balance exercises. I designed the exercise series so that you could do them one after another. This approach allows for an active recovery period. This saves you time and builds a cardiovascular component into your program.

Under the Strength Exercises I have listed the prime or main muscles involved in executing the exercise as well as which part of your skeleton gets the most stimulation from the exercise. The three most frequent bone fracture areas (spine, hip, and wrist) are identified. The muscle groups and affected bones are listed under "Targets."

For example, while doing a squat, your muscles at the front of your thighs and your buttocks are the most active and your hip bones are loaded. Your spine gets loaded as you hold your chest forward, hold a weight, or wear a weighted vest while doing your squat.

Use of Affirmations During the Warm Up Exercises

You should use personal affirmations as you go through your Warm Ups to start your session off on the right foot and get yourself into the right frame of mind. An affirmation is a positive personal thought. As you inhale, say to yourself "I am." As you exhale, choose an affirmation to take with you into your workout: "energized"… "balanced" ... "strong" .... "focussed". Now onto your first Warm Up Exercise.

WARM UP 1 – LATERAL LUNGE

STARTING POSITION:

» Stand tall with your feet shoulder width apart.

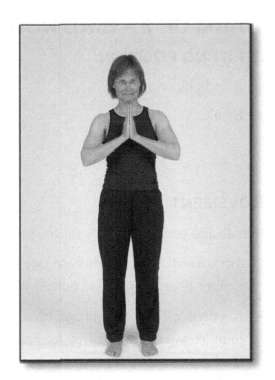

MOVEMENT:

» Take a large step out to the side as you transfer your weight to your right forward foot and heel.

» Keep your feet pointing forward and flat on the floor.

» Sit back behind your right heel and keep your back long, your eyes forward, and your chest elevated.

» Straighten your left leg but do not lock your left knee.

» Return to the standing position and repeat on the other side.

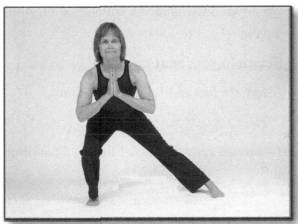

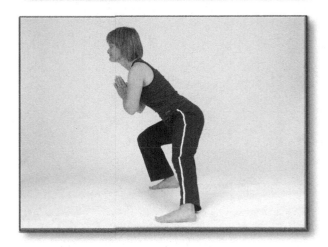

Elite Warm Up Exercises

WARM UP 2 – BIRD NOD

STARTING POSITION:

» Stand tall, palms together.

» Inhale.

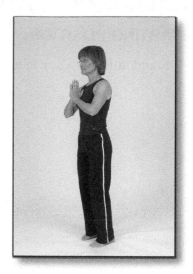

MOVEMENT:

Exhale and gently tighten your lower tummy as you:

» Transfer all your weight onto one leg, keep your knee bent at a twenty-degree angle and extend your arms out to your side.

» Keep your body straight and pivot around your supporting hip joint as you raise your free leg back; simultaneously lower your trunk.

» Go down only as far as you are comfortable and able to keep your hips level.

» Return to your start position.

» Alternate feet until your set is done.

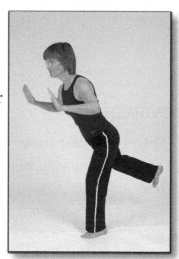

This exercise reminds me of the toy "nodding birds" – hence the name!

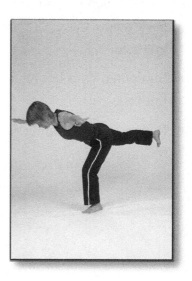

Elite Warm Up Exercises

WARM UP 3 – LUNGE STEPS

STARTING POSITION:

» Place both hands in front of you on a 12-inch high stable step.

» Place one foot back and the other forward close to the step and directly below the front knee.

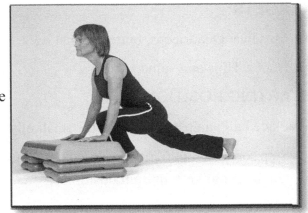

MOVEMENT:

» Press on the step with both hands and maintain the pressure.

» While maintaining your press position on the step, explosively move the back leg to the forward position and the forward leg to the back position in a lunge like fashion.

» Repeat the lunge.

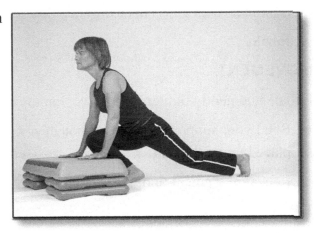

TIP

» Be sure you keep your back straight as you perform this exercise.

Elite Warm Up Exercises

SINGLE LEG WALL SQUAT WITH BALL

TARGETS:

» Muscles: Quadriceps, buttocks, and back.

» Bones: Hips and spine.

STARTING POSITION:

» Place ball against the wall in the small of your back.

» Step forward 4 to 6 inches (approximately a half of your foot length) from your upright position.

» Center one leg under your belly button and raise the other leg and hold it either in front of or behind your supporting leg.

» Stand tall with your hands on your hips.

» Inhale.

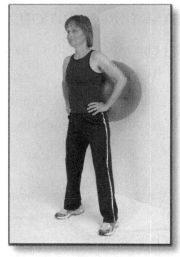

MOVEMENT:

Exhale and gently tighten your lower tummy as you:

» Bend your supporting knee as though you are sitting on a stool placed under the ball.

» Repeat movement until set is completed.

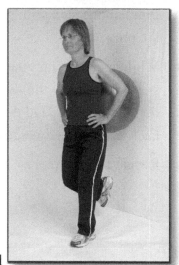

TIP:

» As you squat, the ball will move to your mid- and upper-back region and your weight will be evenly distributed on your heel and forefoot.

» Keep the middle of your knee pointing in the same direction as your second toe.

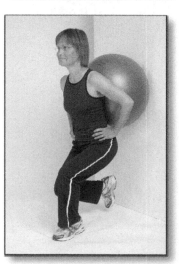

Elite Strength Exercises

BALL T'S

TARGETS:

» Muscles: Neck extensors, spinal extensors, back, shoulders, and buttocks.

» Bones: Spine.

STARTING POSITION:

» Kneel behind ball and mount the ball so that your weight rests on your pelvis when you come forward.

» Tuck your toes under you with your feet shoulder-width apart.

» Arms should rest in front of the ball.

» Inhale.

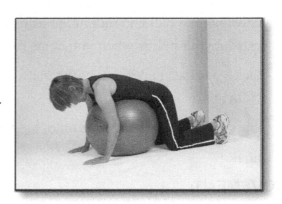

MOVEMENT:

Exhale and gently tighten your lower tummy as you:

» Push forward and extend your torso over the ball.

» Pull your shoulder blades downward and together as you bring your arms out to create a "T" formation.

» Lead with your thumbs and keep your elbows unlocked.

» Keep your head and spine in line.

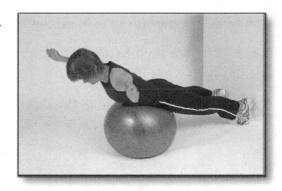

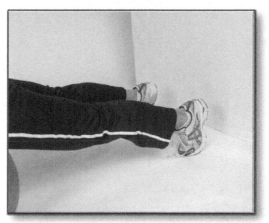

Elite Strength Exercises

BALL M'S

TARGETS:

» Muscles: Neck extensors, spinal extensors, back, shoulders, and buttocks.

» Bones: Spine and hips.

STARTING POSITION:

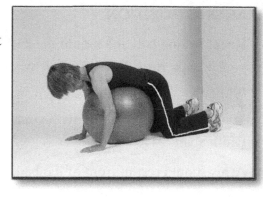

» Kneel behind ball and mount the ball so your weight rests on your pelvis when you come forward.

» Tuck your toes under you with your feet shoulder-width apart.

» Arms should be resting in front of the ball.

» Inhale.

MOVEMENT:

Exhale and gently tighten your lower tummy as you:

» Push forward and extend your torso over the ball.

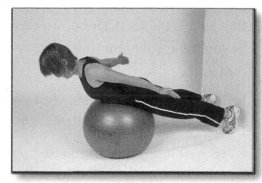

» Pull your shoulder blades downward and together as you bring your arms out to create an "M" formation.

» Lead with your thumbs and keep your elbows unlocked.

» Keep your head and spine in line.

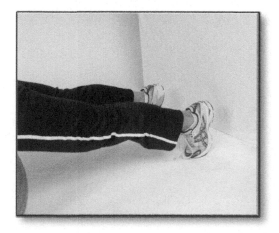

Elite Strength Exercises

BALL Y'S

TARGETS:

» Muscles: Neck extensors, spinal extensors, back, shoulders, and buttocks.

» Bones: Spine and hips.

STARTING POSITION:

» Kneel behind ball and mount the ball so your weight rests on your pelvis when you come forward.

» Tuck your toes under you with your feet shoulder-width apart.

» Arms should be resting in front of the ball.

» Inhale.

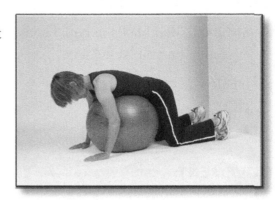

MOVEMENT:

Exhale and gently tighten your lower tummy as you:

» Push forward and extend your torso over the ball.

» Pull your shoulder blades downward and together as you bring your arms out to create a "Y" formation.

» Lead with your thumbs and keep your elbows unlocked.

» Keep your head and spine in line.

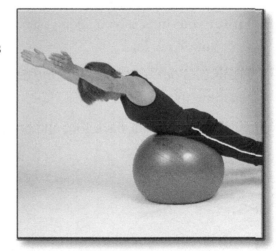

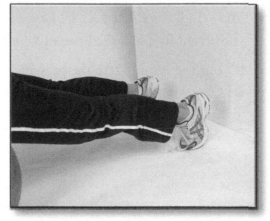

Elite Strength Exercises

WALKING LUNGE WITH WEIGHT

TARGETS:

» Muscles: Hamstrings, buttocks, and quadriceps.

» Bones: Hips, spine, and wrist.

STARTING POSITION:

» Stand tall, dumbbells in both hands and arms either at your side or resting on your shoulders.

» Inhale.

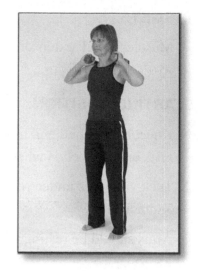

MOVEMENT:

Exhale and gently tighten your lower tummy as you:

» Take a large step forward.

» Lower your hips as you keep your ear, shoulders, and hips in line over your back knee.

» Focus on your back knee coming down toward the floor, but not touching the floor.

» Push off with your back foot and bring that leg up and forward to start the next lunge.

» Repeat movement, alternating legs until set is completed.

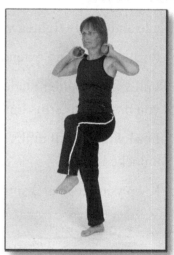

TIPS:

» Both knees should align with corresponding second toe.

» You will have at least six inches of space between the heel of your front foot and the knee of your back leg.

» If your toes do not like the pressure, you may try this exercise wearing running shoes.

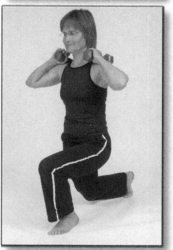

Elite Strength Exercises

STEP UP TO OVERHEAD LIFT

TARGETS:

» Muscles: Shoulders, quadriceps, and buttocks.

» Bones: Hips, spine, and wrist.

STARTING POSITION:

» Stand in front of a step with feet facing forward and shoulder-width apart (begin with a surface that is 4- to 8-inches high).

» Hold dumbbells at shoulder height with your palms facing forward.

» Inhale.

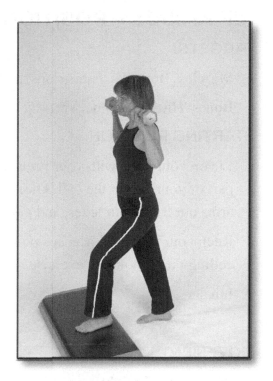

MOVEMENT:

Exhale and gently tighten your lower tummy as you:

» Step-up onto raised surface with one foot.

» Explode up onto the step using your momentum to raise the weights overhead.

» Lower the dumbbells as you lower yourself back to the floor.

» Alternate legs until your set is completed.

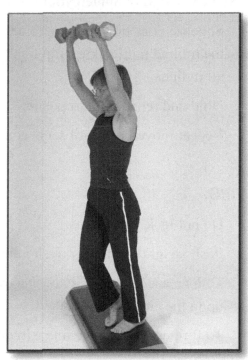

Elite Strength Exercises

HIP RAISES – POSITION A

TARGETS:

» Muscles: Buttocks, hamstrings, and back.

» Bones: Hips and spine.

STARTING POSITION:

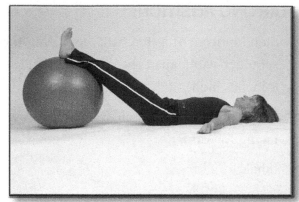

» Lie on your back with your heels and lower part of your leg on the ball, knees slightly bent, arms out from your sides, and palms up.

» Keep your feet and kneecaps pointing to the ceiling throughout the exercise.

» Inhale.

MOVEMENT:

Exhale and gently tighten your lower tummy as you:

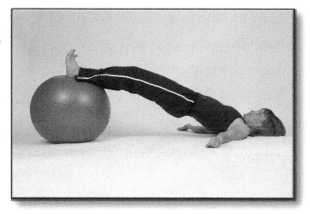

» Squeeze your buttocks and raise your hips off the ground until ankles, hips, and shoulders are all in line.

» Hold and return to start position.

» Repeat movement until set is completed.

TIPS:

» Do not lock your knees.

» Push weight through your shoulder blades and not your neck.

» To increase the intensity of this exercise, place your arms in a "T" or "Y" position, or straight up in the air.

» To further increase the intensity of this exercise, place only your heels on the ball.

Elite Strength Exercises

HIP RAISES – POSITION B

TARGETS:

» Muscles: Buttocks, hamstrings, and back.

» Bones: Hips and spine.

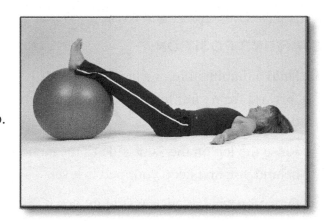

STARTING POSITION:

» Lie on your back with your heels and lower part of your legs on the ball, knees slightly bent, arms out from your sides, and palms up.

» Keep your feet and kneecaps pointing to the ceiling throughout the exercise.

» Inhale.

MOVEMENT:

Exhale and gently tighten your lower tummy as you:

» Squeeze your buttocks and raise your hips off the ground until ankles, hips, and shoulders are all in line.

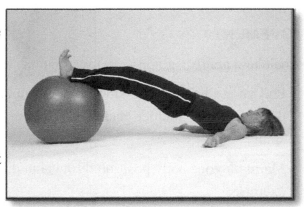

» Roll the ball toward you further raising your hips so that you can draw a line between your shoulders, hips, and knees.

» Return to start position by reversing movement (extend knees until ankles, hips, and shoulders are in line before you lower your hips).

» Repeat movement until set is completed.

TIPS:

» Push weight through your shoulder blades and not your neck.

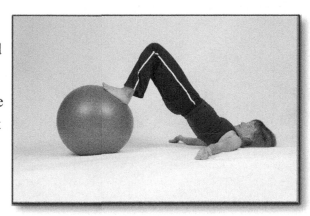

» To increase the intensity of this exercise, place your arms in a "T" or "Y" position, or straight up in the air.

» To further increase the intensity of this exercise, place only your heels on the ball.

Elite Strength Exercises

SINGLE LEG ROW

TARGETS:

» Muscles: Upper back, buttocks, and hamstrings.

» Bones: Hips, spine, and wrist.

STARTING POSITION:

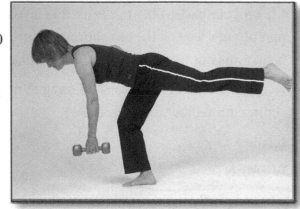

» Hold a dumbbell in one hand and bend forward from your hips with knees bent at a 20 degree angle and butt out.

» Raise the leg on the same side as the dumbbell behind you and keep your pelvis level.

» Drop your weighted arm straight down from your shoulder without locking your elbow.

» Inhale.

MOVEMENT:

Exhale and gently tighten your lower tummy as you:

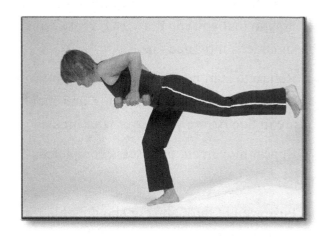

» Pull your elbow to your side simultaneously drawing your shoulder blade towards your spine.

» Maintain your body position throughout the exercise.

» Repeat movement until set is completed.

» Switch sides and repeat.

TIPS:

» Pulling your elbow to body height will reduce stress on the shoulder joint.

Elite Strength Exercises

HIP RAISES – POSITION C

TARGETS:

» Muscles: Hamstrings, buttocks, and back.

» Bones: Hips and spine.

STARTING POSITION:

» Lie on your back with your feet on the side of the ball, knees slightly bent, arms out from your sides and palms up.

» Ball should be immobile.

» Keep your feet and kneecaps pointing to the ceiling throughout the exercise.

» Inhale.

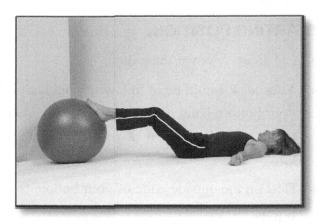

MOVEMENT:

Exhale and gently tighten your lower tummy as you:

» Squeeze buttocks and raise hips off the ground until your shoulder, hips, and knees are in line.

» Hold and return to start position.

» Repeat movement until set is completed.

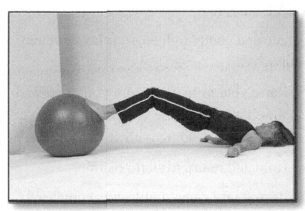

TIPS:

» Push weight through your shoulder blades and not your neck.

Elite Strength Exercises

SIDE LYING LEG LIFTS ON BALL

TARGETS:

» Muscles: Hip abductors.

» Bones: Hips and wrist.

STARTING POSITION:

» Lie sideways over the ball.

» Your legs should be in line with your body, your bottom hand resting on the floor, directly under your shoulder; tuck your elbow into the ball.

» Rest on the outside edge of your bottom foot.

» Inhale.

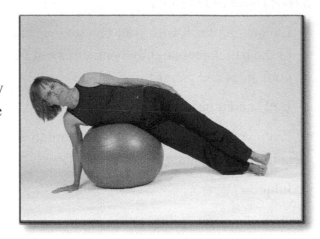

MOVEMENT:

Exhale and gently tighten your lower tummy as you:

» Raise your arm away from your torso and simultaneously raise your top leg to the height of your hip, leading with your heel.

» Hold and return to start position.

» Repeat movement until set is completed.

» Switch sides and repeat.

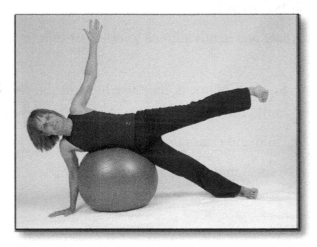

VARIATION:

» Raise leg as above but hand rests on ball in front of body for added stability.

Elite Strength Exercises

PULLOVER ON BALL (WITH TWO WEIGHTS)

TARGETS:

» Muscles: Back, hips, and spinal extensors.

» Bones: Spine, hips, and wrists.

STARTING POSITION:

» Carefully sit on the ball – you can stabilize it by resting your weighted hand on it.

» Once you are sitting on the ball bring the weight against your chest.

» Walk your feet forward while at the same time lowering your body.

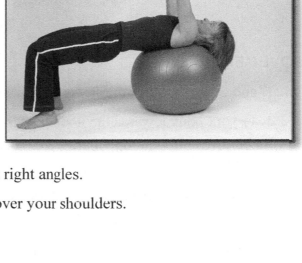

» Once the ball is resting under your upper shoulder blades and head, lift your hips until your torso and thighs are in a table-top position (buttocks and thighs in line with shoulders) and knees bent at right angles.

» Raise the weights towards the ceiling directly over your shoulders.

» Inhale.

MOVEMENT:

Exhale and gently tighten your lower tummy as you:

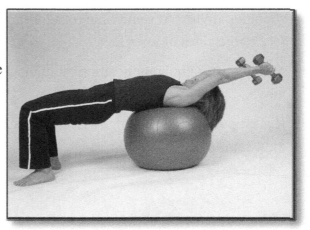

» Move the weights overhead until your arms are beside your ears.

» Keep your buttocks squeezed. Keep hips in line with your shoulders and knees.

» Slowly return weights to the starting position.

» Repeat movement until set is completed.

TIP:

» Keep your lower ribs down as you raise your arms behind you.

Elite Strength Exercises

PUSH UP WITH A TWIST

TARGETS:

» Muscles: Chest, triceps, deep abdominals, and back

» Bones: Wrists, spine, and hips

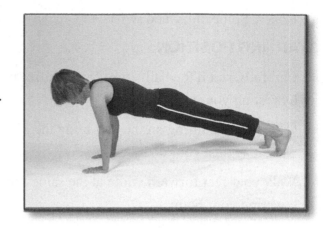

STARTING POSITION:

» Place your hands and feet a little wider than shoulder-width apart in a full-plank position.

» Inhale.

MOVEMENT:

Exhale and gently tighten your lower tummy as you:

» Lower your body towards the floor, bending your elbows until your upper arms are parallel to the floor.

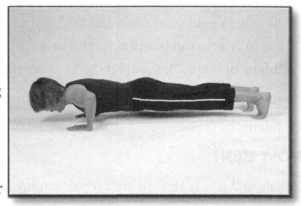

» Push body up away from floor by straightening your arms.

» Using the momentum, transfer to an open position balancing on single hand with your shoulder at 90°. At same time rotate from your toes to the sides of your feet.

» Maintain straight body position throughout the move.

» Repeat push-up alternating twist left to right until set is completed.

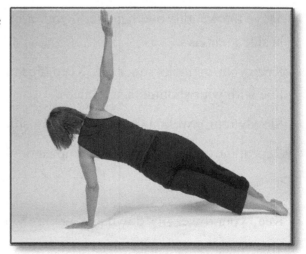

Elite Strength Exercises

LATERAL LUNGE WITH BICEPS CURL

TARGETS:

» Muscles: Biceps, buttocks, quadriceps, and hips.

» Bones: Spine and wrists.

STARTING POSITION:

» Stand tall.

» Hold dumbbells with palms facing thighs.

» Inhale.

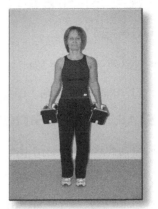

MOVEMENT:

Exhale and gently tighten your lower tummy as you:

» Take a large step to the left, shifting your body weight over your left hip as you lunge (weights should be on either side of left leg).

» Sit back behind your left heel and keep your back long, your eyes forward, and your chest open.

» Push off with your left leg and return to start position.

» As you begin your biceps curl, move palms from their start position, facing thighs, to palms facing forward.

» Bring the weights to your shoulders.

» Hold and return to start position.

» Repeat lunge and biceps curl, alternating sides until set is completed.

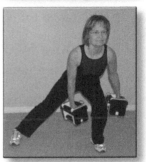

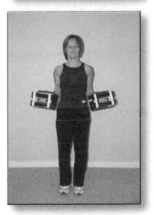

TIP:

» During the lunge, be sure to keep your feet facing forward, your knees in line with toes, your chest lifted.

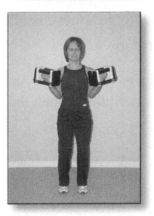

Elite Strength Exercises

TRICEPS EXTENSION ON BALL – POSITION A

TARGETS:

» Muscles: Triceps, shoulders, buttocks, and hamstrings.

» Bones: Wrists, hips, and spine.

STARTING POSITION:

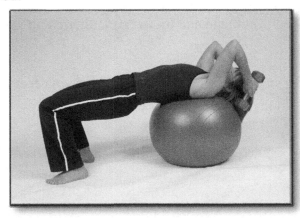

» Carefully sit on the ball – you can stabilize it by resting your weighted hand on it.

» Once you are sitting on the ball bring the weight against your chest.

» Walk your feet forward while at the same time lowering your body.

» Once the ball is resting under your upper shoulder blades and head, lift your hips until your torso and thighs are in a table-top position (buttocks and thighs in line with shoulders), knees bent at right angles.

» Arms are straight and raised slightly higher than shoulder height (weights are in line with your eyes/forehead).

» Inhale.

MOVEMENT:

Exhale and gently tighten your lower tummy as you:

» Bend your elbow, lowering the weights.

» Hold and return to start position.

» Repeat movement until set is completed.

TIPS:

» Keep your shoulders, upper arms, and body still throughout the exercise.

» Do not lock your elbows.

Elite Strength Exercises

TRICEPS EXTENSION ON BALL – POSITION B

TARGETS:

» Muscles: Triceps, shoulders, buttocks, and hamstrings.

» Bones: Wrists, hips, and spine.

STARTING POSITION:

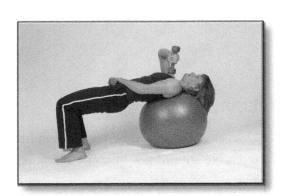

» Carefully sit on the ball – you can stabilize it by resting your weighted hand on it.

» Once you are sitting on the ball bring the weight against your chest.

» Walk your feet forward while at the same time lowering your body.

» Once the ball is resting under your upper shoulder blades and head, lift your hips until your torso and thighs are in a table-top position (buttocks and thighs in line with shoulders), knees bent at 90°.

» Once the ball is resting under your upper shoulder blades and head, lift your hips until your torso and thighs are in a table-top position (buttocks and thighs in line with shoulders), knees bent at a 90 degree angle.

» One arm is bent and resting over pelvis. Other arm is straight and raised in line over the shoulder. Your thumb should be pointing toward the opposite shoulder.

» Inhale.

MOVEMENT:

Exhale and gently tighten your lower tummy as you:

» Bend your elbow, lowering your forearm across your chest to your opposite shoulder.

» Hold and return to start position.

» Repeat until set is completed

» Repeat movement with alternate arm.

TIPS:

» Keep your shoulders, upper arms, and body still throughout the exercise.

» Do not lock your elbow.

Elite Strength Exercises

SQUAT JUMPS

TARGETS:

» Muscles: Calves, quadriceps, buttocks, and hips.

» Bones: Spine.

STARTING POSITION:

» Stand with feet shoulder width apart.

» Inhale and activate your abdominals as you lower yourself into a squat, bend at the hips and knees, keep your eyes forward.

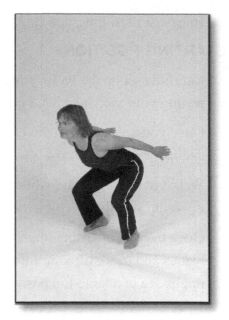

MOVEMENT:

Exhale gently tighten your lower tummy as you:

» Jump, exploding up.

» Extend ankles, knees, and hips in a straight line.

» Absorb the jump by allowing your knees to bend as you land.

» Repeat until set is completed.

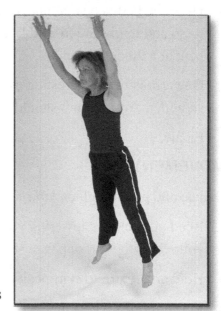

SPECIAL NOTE:

» Due to the increased compression forces upon landing, this exercise should not be done by individuals who are at a high fracture risk.

Elite Strength Exercises

ABDOMINAL ACTIVATION LEG DROPS – ADVANCED

TARGETS:

» Muscles: Transverse abdominus.

» Bones: Spine.

STARTING POSITION:

» Lie on your back, legs together with hips and knees at a 90 degree angle.

» Place a small rolled towel in the small of your back (roll should be the width and depth of the of your hand).

» Inhale.

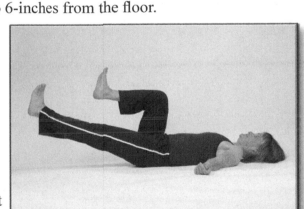

MOVEMENT:

Exhale and gently tighten your lower tummy as you:

» Slowly lower and straighten left leg 4-inches to 6-inches from the floor.

» Right leg remains in the start position.

» Return left leg to start position and repeat using right leg.

» Repeat movement alternating legs until set is completed.

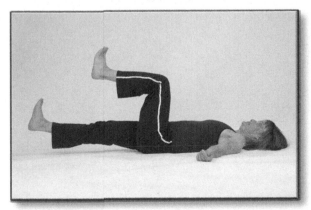

TIPS:

» If you are unable to keep your abdominals tight for the full set, then return to the start position, take a short rest, and resume the set.

» The lower you drop your leg the greater the challenge.

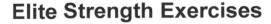

Elite Strength Exercises

16. Elite Level Balance Exercises

Balance is a critical component of your exercise program. Balance becomes increasingly important as our bones age and become more fragile. We use our balance to keep us from falls that could lead to a fracture.

Increased balance allows you to be more independent and confident and can greatly affect the quality of your life. The more balanced you are when you perform day-to-day activities, the more likely you are to be active in life.

The balance exercises in this chapter have been developed for people who are at a Low fracture risk. If you have a high fracture risk, please refer back to the Beginner or Active Level programs (in Chapters 10 and 12). If you have a moderate fracture risk, please refer back to the Athletic Level balance exercises (in Chapter 14).

These balance exercises will make you more stable and will have a direct impact on reducing your fracture risk. With practice, your balance will improve. Follow these instructions when you are performing your balance training:

» Choose among the exercises listed that challenge you.

» Make sure that you can hold your position for at least 10 seconds.

» Mix up the exercises from week to week for variety.

» Do a total of 3 to 5 minutes of balance training each session.

» Keep safety in mind by practicing your balance exercises in a safe location, such as a corner of a room with a sturdy chair in front of you for support.

» Maintain an athletic stance as discussed in Chapter 4.

At the Elite Level, the jump landings are done on one foot. This not only maximizes the balance requirement, but also the impact through the skeleton.

The balance exercises for Elite are quite advanced and should be practiced only under the following guidelines:

» Before you begin you want to power up your posture with an athletic stance!

» This series of drills involves jumps. It is geared towards the elite athlete with low bone density or who is on a prevention program and is not suitable for clients with osteoporosis.

» You should have mastered all the exercises in the Elite Strength training program.

» Ensure that your jumping form is perfect before you attempt any of the exercises in this chapter.

AROUND THE CLOCK

Imagine you are standing in the center of a large clock with your feet shoulder width apart.

» Start by jumping forward onto both feet.

» Hold for a count of two seconds and then jump back to the start position.

» Progress to jumping to the left and then to the right (3 o'clock and 9 o'clock).

» Jump to 10, 2, 9, and 8 o'clock returning to the start position each time.

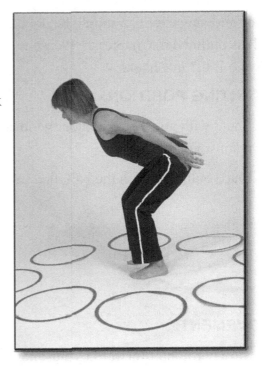

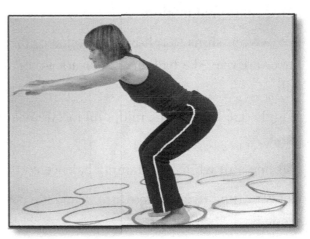

Elite Balance Exercises

THREE POINT BALANCE ON BALL

The following exercise should be done using the correct sized ball as outlined in Chapter 2. Please review "Safely Using a Physio Ball" in Chapter 4.

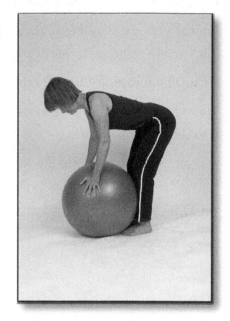

STARTING POSITION:

» Stand with your feet shoulder width apart; roll the ball against your shins.

» Place both hands on the ball directly under your shoulders.

MOVEMENT:

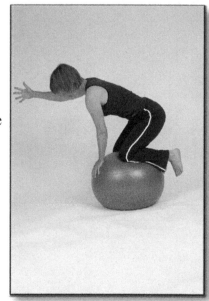

» Slowly roll ball forward by pushing off with your feet in a slow, controlled motion.

» Allow your shins to follow the motion of the ball until your knees are over the ball and hands are on the front part of the ball.

» Wiggle one hand to the midpoint location between both hands.

» Lift one arm while maintaining balance on ball.

» Repeat lifting the opposite arm. Hold the pose for up to 10 seconds.

» A more advanced 3-point position is to lift your leg as illustrated in the photo to the immediate right.

» Do both sides holding each leg for up to 10 seconds.

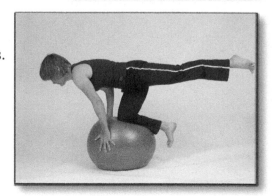

Elite Balance Exercises

KNEELING ON BALL

The following exercise should be done using the correct sized ball as outlined in Chapter 2. Please review "Safely Using a Physio Ball" in Chapter 4.

STARTING POSITION:

» Stand with your feet shoulder width apart; roll the ball against your shins.

» Place both hands on the ball directly under your shoulders.

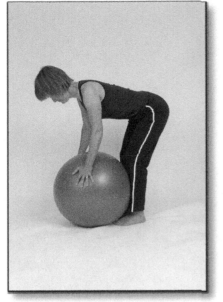

MOVEMENT:

» Slowly roll ball forward by pushing off with your feet in a slow, controlled motion.

» Allow your shins to follow the motion of the ball until your knees are over the ball and hands are on the front part of the ball.

» Roll the ball further forward and bring your shins to rest over top of the ball (your toes should be able to touch the ball if you pulled them in.)

» Hold for up to 30 seconds.

» Return back to 4-point on the ball before dismounting.

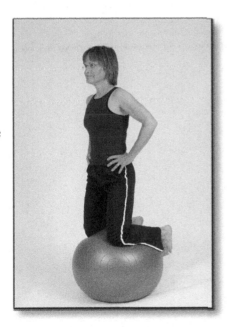

Elite Balance Exercises

Follow Margaret

SIGN UP FOR MY ONLINE NEWSLETTER

I publish an online newsletter and I would love to see you subscribe to it. It is delivered to your email inbox. The newsletter is informative and covers a wide range of health topics and tips – not just bone health!

Visit **www.melioguide.com/enews** and sign up. I do not SPAM or share my email list with other parties. You can unsubscribe from the email list at any time by clicking on the unsubscribe link inside any of the emails that I send to you.

OTHER BOOKS I HAVE PUBLISHED

Besides Exercise for Better Bones, I have published two other books.

Strengthen Your Core

Strengthen Your Core is for anyone who wants a safe and effective core exercise program. The program uses Plank and Side Plank poses to improve posture, enhance performance, and strengthen from head to toe.

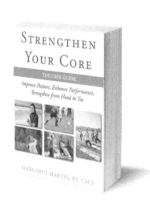

The book discusses the theory behind core strength so that you will have a solid understanding of how to build and develop core strength. Detailed descriptions with photos are provided for each of the poses.

Four levels are provided to meet your needs: Beginner, Active,

Athletic and Elite. Strengthen Your Core is available in Kindle or print formats.

Yoga for Better Bones

Yoga for Better Bones is a must for yoga practitioners and teachers who want to make sure that their yoga poses are safe for someone with osteoporosis, osteopenia/low bone density.

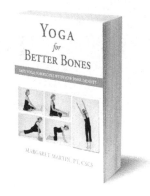

The book shows how to modify popular yoga poses that potentially put your bones at risk of fracture. The book is illustrated with clear photos and images.

Yoga for Better Bones is available in print format and soon will be available for your Kindle.

Research Reference List

I have indicated in Chapters 1 and 3 where I have used specific studies or articles. These studies are noted below. The number next to the article corresponds with the number identified in Chapters 1 and 3.

Chapter 1 – Welcome: Reference List

1. Zehnacker CH, Effects of Weighted Exercises on Bone Mineral Density in Post Menopausal Women: A Systemic Review, Journal of Geriatric Physical Therapy 2007

2. Kohrt WM et al. Physical Activity and Bone Health. ACSM Position Stand. Medicine and Science in Sports and Exercise 36 (11): 1985-1996, 2004

3. Kerr D, Morton A, Dick I. Et al. Exercise effects on bone mass in post-menopausal women are site-specific and load-dependent. J Bone Min Res. 1996;11:218-225

4. Kannus P, Haapasalo H, Sandelo M, Sievanen H, Pasanen M, Heinonen A, Oja P, Vuori I. Effect of starting age of physical activity on bone mass in the dominant arm of tennis and squash players. Ann Intern Med 1995; 123:27-31

5. Bassey J, Ramsdale S. Increases in femoral bone density in young women following high-impact exercise. Osteoporosis Int. 1994;4:72-75

6. Rubin CT, Lanyon LE. Regulation of bone mass by mechanical strain magnitude. Calcif Tissue Int 1985; 37:411-7

7. Pruitt LA, Jackson RD, Bartels RL, et al. Weight-training effects on bone mineral density in early postmenopausal women. J Bone Miner Res 1992;7:179-85

8. Martyn-StJames M, Carroll S. Meta-analysis of walking for preservation of bone mineral density in postmenopausal women. Bone. 2008 Sep 43(3):521-31

9. Kemmler W, Engelke K, von Stengel S, Weineck J, et al. Long-Term Four-Year Exercise Has A Positive Effect On Menopausal Risk factors: The Erlangen Fitness Osteoporosis Prevention Study. J of Strength and Conditioning Research, 2007, 21(1), 232-239

10. Canada Task Force for Preventive Health Care Clinical Practice Guidelines - DXA Guidelines Cheung AM et al. CMAJ 2004;170(11):1665-1667

Chapter 3 – Bone and Body Basics: Reference List

1. Sinaki and Mikkelson Postmenopausal Spinal Osteoporosis: Flexion versus Extension Exercises Arch Phys Med Rehabil Vol 65, October, 1984

2. Wilson SE. Development of a Model to Predict the Compressive Forces on the Spine Associated with Age-related Vertebral Fractures. Cambridge, Mass: Massachusetts Institute of Technology; 1994

3. Gokkaya O NK, et al. Reduced aerobic capacity in patients with severe osteoporosis: a cross sectional study. Eur J Phys Rehabil Med. 2008 Jun;44(2):141-7.

4. "Fast Facts" NOF, January 1, 2009 http://www.nof.org/osteoporosis/diseasefacts.htm

5. Ross, P et al Pre-existing Fractures and Bone Mass Predict Vertebral Fracure Incidence in Women, Annals of Internal Med. 114 (11): 919-923 1991

6. Huntoon EA, Schmidt CK, in patients who engage in back-extensor strengthening exercises. Mayo Clin Proc. abstract 2008 Jan;83(1):54-7

7. Betz S. Modifying Pilates for Clients With Osteoporosis, *Inner Idea 2007*

The following are research studies and articles that I have reviewed in preparation of this guide. They do not correspond to specific sections of the guide. I have broken them down by topical area.

Exercise: Additional Reference Material

1. Kerr D, Ackland T, Maslen B, et al. Resitance training over 2 years increases bone mass in calcium-replete postmenauposal women. *J Bone Miner Res* 2001;16:175-181

2. Kerr D, Morton A, Dick I. Et al. Exercise effects on bone mass in post-menopausal women are site-specific and load-dependent. *J Bone Min Res.* 1996;11:218-225

3. Sherrington C, Lord SR, Herbert RD. A randomized controlled trial of weight-bearing versus non-weight-bearing exercise for improving physical ability after usual care for hip fracture. *Arch Phys Med Rehabil.* 2004;85:710-716

4. Krolner B, Toft B. Vertebral bone loss:anunheeded side effect of therapeutic bed rest. *Clin Sci.* 1983; 64:537-540

5. Heinomen A, Kannus P, Sievanen H, et al. Randomized controlled trial of effect of high-impact exercise on selected risk factors for osteoporotic fractures. *Lancet.* 1996;348:1343-1347

6. Woolf I, Van Croonenborg JJ, Kemper HCG, et al. The effects of exercise training programs on bone mass: a meta-analysis of published controlled trials in pre and postmenopausal women. Osteoporosis Int. 1999;9:1-12.

7. Layne JE, Nelson ME. The effects of progressive resistance training on bone density: as review. *Med Sci Sports Exerc.* 1999;31:25-30

8. Frost HM. Why do marathon runners have less bone than weight lifters? A vital-

biomechanical view and explanation. *Bone*. 1997;20:183-189

9. Petit MA, McKay HA, MacKelvie KJ, et al. A randomized school-based jumping intervention confers site and maturity-specific benefits on bone structural properties in girls: a hip structural analysis study. *J Bone Miner Res*. 2002:363-372

10. Winchester JB, et al., Static Stretching Impairs Sprint Performance in Collegiate Track and Field Athletes, *Journal of Strength and Conditioning Research*, Vol. 22, No. 1, January 2008 pgs. 13 – 18

11. Rob D Herbert, Michael Gabriel, Effects of stretching before and after exercising on muscle soreness and risk of injury: systematic review. *BMJ* 2002;325: 46

12. Rikli RE and Jones JC, Senior Fitness Test Manual. Champaign: *Human Kinetics* 2001

13. Ott, S. Bone Density in Athletes <http://depts.washington.edu/bonebio/bonStrength/exercise/sports.html> February 1, 2008

14. Crews L, Yoga for seniors. Inner Idea, January 2007

15. Bailey, DA et al. A six year longitudinal study of the relationship of physical activity to Bone Mineral Accrual in growing children: The Univ. of Saskatchewan Bone Mineral Accrual Study. *J Bone Miner Res* 1999; 14(10): 1672-1679

16. Borer, K.T, "Physical activity in the prevention and amelioration of osteoporosis in women", *Sports Medicine*, 35(9), pp 779-830, 2005

17. Ari Heinonen et al., *Lancet* 1996

18. Chubak J. et al. Effect of Exercise on Bone Mineral Density and Lean Mass in Postmenopausal Women

19. *Med Sci Sports Exerc*. 2006; 38(7):1236-1244

20. Asikainen TM et al. "Exercise for Health for Early Postmenopausal Women", *Sports Medicine* 2004, 34(11), pp 753-778

21. Evans, William J et al. "AstroFit", The Free Press, 2002

Balance: Additional Reference Material

1. FallProof!: A Comprehensive Balance and Mobility Training Program, Rose Debra J.; Champaign: Human Kinetics, 2003
2. Sinaki M et al. *Osteoporosis Int.* Balance disorder and increased risk of falls in osteoporosis and kyphosis: significance of kyphotic posture and muscle strength. 2005 Aug; 16(8):1004-10.
3. TE Howe, L Rochester, A Jackson, PMH Banks, VA Blair. Exercise for improving balance in older people. *Cochrane Database of Systematic Reviews* 2007 Issue 4

Core Exercises: Additional Reference Material

1. McGill, S. Ultimate Back Fitness and Performance 3rd Edition Backfitpro Inc. 2006

Posture: Additional Reference Material

1. Lewis CB. The Relationship Between Posture and Psychological Variables in Students Age 18 - 25. *Oregon Free Press.* 1983.
2. Paul Hodges Lumbopelvic Motor Control: Clinical techniques in motor control training for lumbopelvic pain. Hamilton, ON Feb. 7, 2009
3. Meeks, SM, OSTEOPOROSIS: A Comprehensive Treatment Strategy Level 1 by Sara M. Meeks, PT, MS, GCS. San Francisco, CA 2001